HOME-CENTERED
HEALTH CARE

Home-Centered Health Care

The Populist Transformation
of the American Health Care System

Mike Magee, MD

Library of Congress Cataloging-in-Publication Data
Magee, Mike.
Home-Centered Health Care/Mike Magee, MD
160p. 20.32x12.7cm

ISBN 1-889793-22-1

Manufactured in Canada
First Edition

To America's
informal family caregivers,
who deserve our thanks, gratitude,
and undying support

Contents

PROLOGUE

From Yellow Pages to Health Care Carousel

WILLIAM L. MINNIX, JR.

America needs a vision for health care and Dr. Mike Magee offers one! He uses a metaphor from a childhood trip to the World's Fair where he reflects on the "Carousel of Progress"—a creative walk through time about the progressive evolution of science and technology as applied to our everyday lives, bringing to life a vision of the possible.

In *Home Centered Health Care*, Mike Magee describes a vision of a "Carousel of Health" where the alignments of powerful forces are redirecting our collective consciousness toward a transformational era that leads to health—and continuous progress toward it—even the experience of dying and death as the natural end to this bio-mystical phenomena called the human life cycle.

If Mike Magee shows us a vision for the "Carousel of Health" what do we have now? The metaphor of a "Yellow Pages of Services" comes to mind. Yes, our country is flooded with myriad service providers—thousands of pages of directories of them. Some officially sanctioned, approved, inspected, regulated and patched together in various planned options with multiple plans for payments. Other services are often informal and untold numbers of elderly, disabled and vulnerable people rely on these every day to cope with chronic conditions.

I remember years ago taking my father to his physician who was part of a prestigious medical center. As we entered the grand lobby to the office suite, I noticed what appeared to be a paid caregiver wheeling an elderly man in a chair up to the marquee. The caregiver was trying to discern from her impaired client the name of the physician or service to be visited. There was no person in sight to call on for information.

My father and I easily found the information we needed, proceeded to the elevator and continued our quest to the doctor's office. When we returned some half-hour later, the old man and his caregiver were still at the marquee trying to decipher what to do, where to go and who to see. In the midst of a splendid maze of facilities, with access to comprehensive prenatal to terminal care, delivered by some of the world's best trained professionals—there was a lost soul and his caregiver! An all too common experience, I would bet.

In the richest country in the world when it comes to health care talent, money and services, why do we have difficulty producing the best results? Why are services fragmented? Why are there millions of uninsured? Why is Medicaid going broke? Why are there too many nursing homes and not enough services to help people in need stay at home? Why are there parts of this Yellow Pages array of services awash in money and other aspects grossly under-funded? Why do we have outstanding emergency rooms and very little proactive health promotion? Why do impaired elderly wander the halls of health-care-aplenty with their caregivers and not know how to get help?

I've asked these questions of many Washington policy wonks. The *one* consistent answer might surprise you! Would you guess lack of money? No, most believe there is ample money in the system to assure an excellent health care that is accessible and affordable to all. Greed and control? Many say health care is, after all, big business and nobody wants to lose market share. Yet, health care has perpetually rebalanced itself as needs, wants and financing have changed. The market eventually gets what it wants in our democratic entrepreneurial economy. Lack of political will? Yes, a factor. The great society plan of the 1960's was our last domestic vision that enjoyed political leadership and support. Attempts in the 1990's for political leadership on health care reform met with huge resistance largely based on a flawed process for public debate and a vision likened (fairly or unfairly) to a socialist plot where choice, freedom and privacy would be compromised. So, burned political children rightly fear the fire.

While all of these guesses carry a measure of truth, the *ONE* consistent answer is *lack of vision and planning*. That's where Mike Magee enters the picture with his vision for *Home Centered Health Care*.

This book is a picture of the future—the Carousel we can see—of what healthy, affordable and ethical health care can be. It outlines our *alignment* of phenomena that create a new era that the masses want to move toward because it appeals to all our basic, common sense and self- interests, and common good instincts.

On Dr. Magee's Carousel of Health, we can see that all of us, unless brain impaired, are capable of dealing responsibly with facts and knowledge in the management of our health. The Carousel showcases consumers, within the context of a place he or she calls home where people live every day. In this place called home, technology provides information, feedback and services at chair side, fireside or bedside—like technology provides entertainment. No more wandering the halls of medical wonderland.

The Carousel shows how the consumer's support systems of family, friends and neighbors can be supported in their natural state. No more zoos—just natural habitats.

The Magee Carousel aligns the financing to let money follow the person and not the provider. This shift alone transforms the business paradigm, opening us to new possibilities for products and services, when and where people need them.

By focusing on the *home*, the ethical playing field is leveled. The technology can be made available to all, in equal doses. Thus, appealing to our sense of justice and mercy because accessibility issues virtually vanish and the economics are dramatically changed in the consumer's favor—even the modest-income consumer.

And, finally, the politics are fully aligned: A system that consumers control, in which they have choices, through which they manage their lives better, based on contemporary knowledge and reinforcing their support mechanisms, and is, therefore, at last, affordable!

Home Center Health Care is the Carousel of Progress as envisioned through a true prophet, Dr. Mike Magee. It is time to embrace such a vision. All the dynamics are coming into alignment. His vision appeals to all of us because it helps us see it—and it makes sense. It is a vision of the possible. It is populist transformation—consistent with the best of the American spirit.

William L. Minnix, Jr., D.Min
President and CEO
The American Association of
Homes and Services for the Aging

1.

Overview

As a weekly media commentator on health care issues, I am often asked for my opinion on where our health care system is headed. I have the advantage of being able to share perspectives with a wide range of thinkers in the health care arena—and their opinions on what needs to be done about our health care system cover the entire spectrum of possibilities. Clearly, there is no single perfect set of answers.

Nor is there enough space in this book to offer all the possible scenarios for the future as they relate to the many topics we have covered—from health insurance reform to end-of-life care.

Still, I think the diverse dots that make up the current thinking in health care can be connected—and that a new vision is beginning to emerge. After more than 30 years of observing health care and thinking about what's possible, some things seem undeniable. And I notice that increasingly, voices from disparate sectors and schools of thought are coalescing around these fundamental principles.

With that said, let me lay out what I believe are several general factors and trends that are defining our health care future, and what I believe is the most likely destination they are taking us—toward a new paradigm of care.

The first, and most important, factor is that we are aging

as a society. We must acknowledge that this demographic change will profoundly impact health care as we know it today. Part of that change involves moving from three-generation to four- and five-generation family complexity.[1]

Faced with a complex health care system and the new reality of aging and chronic disease, a vast population of informal caregivers (now present in 25 percent of American families) is on the rise. They are educated, motivated, and involved with health care decisions. They represent a populist force that increasingly questions the status quo.[2]

Recognizing this rising force and the changing dynamics of the patient-physician relationship, physicians have moved from paternalism to partnership, and are moving from individual to team-support models.[3]

At the same time, the medical community is realizing that its infrastructure is not ideally suited for the demands this aging society will put on the health care system. There is, simply put, minimal time and space left in the doctors' offices for preventive care. Our outpatient office-based delivery system is not ideally suited for the rigors of the future.[4]

Combined, these forces point the system toward a logical solution: Properly supported and validated by physicians and nurses with education, behavioral modification, early diagnosis and screening, most care decisions and care functions will increasingly take place in the home. We can call this new paradigm home-centered health care.[5]

I believe the concept of home-centered health care will grow rapidly in coming years, and it will lead to the transformation of informal caregivers into designated home health managers and to their inclusion more formally into the physician-led, often nurse-directed health care team. In this new paradigm, health care teams will coordinate both clinical and educational continuums under physician oversight. Most educational leadership will be delegated by physicians to nurses and other caring professionals who will maintain 24/7-contact with home health managers through virtual health networks.

The virtual health networks will be here soon, thanks to incredible advances in technology. Visionary thinkers in health care technology—ranging from corporate giants such as Intel and Philips Inc. to small, entrepreneurial start-ups—are working today below the radar screen on amazing devices that will revolutionize care and make true networks possible.[6] Those applications will advantage our expanding information highways, built on the backs of digital cable and wireless WiMax installations, which are now reaching the critical mass necessary to connect the people to the people caring for the people.[7,8]

The current surge of private technology investment in home health will outfit homes with pervasive motion/location sensors, vital signs monitoring, blood and imaging diagnostics, intelligence analytic software, personalized prompter coaching interfaces, and Internet data transfer to care networks—functionally bringing the virtual care team and its resources into the home and obviating the need for most office visits and many hospitalizations.[9]

As technology and demographics lead us inexorably toward this new paradigm, the health care financing system will be forced to keep pace. Health insurance will go universal, be portable, and involve multi-year commitments. Health insurers will reimburse physicians fairly for management of teams and oversight of complex databases and will offer incentives for home health managers by providing lower premiums to families who deliver measurably positive health outcomes and effective prevention and screening across the multi-generation family divide.

Pharmaceutical and device companies will invest in consumer education and behavioral modification, early diagnosis and prevention, and a new business model built around home-centered health solutions. Health information highways will be home-centric; that is, begin in the home, extend out to the caregivers, and loop back to the home, rather than the other way around. A continuous robust stream of data will flow out electronically, and 24/7 analysis and coaching will flow back in, in the other direction.[10]

At the end of the day, caring will re-center in the home, where compassion and personalization reside. Here, caring will integrate mind, body, and spirit; focus on wellness and functionality; integrate and prioritize resources along the four- or five-generation family divide; and tailor care to the unique cultural and social needs of family members. On the one hand, adherence to mutually agreed-upon care plans will better manage chronic diseases using the principles of palliative care.[11] On the other, lifespan planning records will attempt to get ahead of the disease curve and delay or completely eliminate chronic disease in future generations.[12]

Homes will look to their communities for value grounding, integrated social systems, and resources if overwhelmed by complexity. Physicians, nurses, and other members of the care teams will advocate for these changes because they make sense and are the only reasonable way to manage the cost and quality demands of global aging societies.

It all may sound a bit futuristic, but the elements of this new paradigm of care are either here now or soon will be. And it will become a reality, thanks to the persistent demands of millions of Americans who make up a consumer empowerment movement that I believe already has built an unstoppable momentum. We might think of the coming transition in health care as a kind of populist uprising—led by consumers who now possess the critical combination of enlightenment, empowerment, and personal motivation needed to assert control over their own health care futures.

Much work remains to be done before this vision of health care will be fully embraced. Some sectors of our health care system continue to cling to the silos of yesterday—in financing, in education, in technology—believing the health space to be segregated from the rest of our lives. But if trends continue to play out as they have recently, the keepers of the silos will soon face head on the force of millions of consumers who demand change. Those consumers will be reinforced by financial, technology, and entertainment sectors anxious to enter the health care space and sharing three strategic resources—vast financial assets, remarkable expertise in information technologies, and a well-established position already in consumers homes.[13]

As for traditional health care leaders, we must embrace new partners and listen to the people and follow their lead— for after all, it's their health and their health care system. Why not strive for excellence in both?

2.

Health Populism and Colliding Megatrends

Some two and a half years ago, I launched the weekly webcast program, Health Politics (www.Health-Politics.org). The goal was simple: using aggressive new media advocacy, simultaneously support the information needs of the people and the people who care for the people. As we approached our 100th anniversary show and were wondering what subject would be appropriate, I received several e-mails questioning whether Health Politics was an appropriate title for the program. I decided to devote our 100th program to answering the question, "Why Health Politics?"

I quickly realized that this would require answering two questions: First, "What is health?" and second, "What is politics?" For me, it was easier to define what health is not, than what it is. Health is not the health care system. Health is not the elimination of disease. Health is not science and technology. And health is not intervention in all its varied shapes and sizes. Health is a state of wellbeing that involves mind, body, and spirit. Health is well reflected in the eyes of a mother who gazes down on her newborn baby and hopes and prays that her little girl will one day have the opportunity to reach her full human potential. Health includes the individual, family, community, and societal support services and encouragement that would turn that potential into reality.

Health is, as Gro Brundtland said from the global platform of the World Health Organization in 1998, "part goodness and part fairness." "Goodness" in the sense that our professionals are well trained and qualified; our institutions well outfitted and safe; our processes engineered to perfection; our teamwork a reflection of training and excellent communication. "Fairness" in the sense that these skills and capabilities are fairly and equitably distributed to the broadest population possible.[1]

Now for the second question, "What is politics?" For some, politics is an apparatus of government, fundamentally top-down and elitist. A few govern the multitude. But for others, politics is the power to support the needs of individuals, families, communities, and society. For these, politics is bottom-up and populist.

But is health political? Clearly the answer is yes. First, the social determinants of health—employment, housing, transportation—are themselves political. Second, health is multifactorial and integrated. For example, clean water— which is vital to health—is affected by agricultural, energy, and urban policy. Third, health involves critical resources that are unequally distributed. Fourth, most now agree that health is more than a market commodity and is increasingly understood as a human right. And finally, health clearly intersects at the crossroads of economic, social, and political theory.[2]

So once again, in the spirit of full disclosure: For me health is a human right; politics is about the people; and health politics is, in fact, health populism.

Within that context, let us look in greater detail at five megatrends that I have been following for over two decades, which are increasingly colliding, synergizing, and accelerating each other. Together they are releasing a wave of transformational forces that will ensure the near-term actualization of a new approach to health care in the United States.

The first trend, of course, is aging. Approximately 50

percent of all 60-year-olds in the United States today have a parent alive. This means that the four-generation American family is commonplace.[3] By the year 2050, more than 1 million Americans will be over 100. This means that the five-generation family will be commonplace. Thus the three-generation family is rapidly being supplanted by the four- and five-generation family with enormous implications for multigenerational health management complexity.[4]

Approximately 25 percent of these complex U.S. families have an informal family caregiver in place. 85 percent of these caregivers are family members, and almost all are third-generation women, aged 45 to 65.[5] They are simultaneously managing parents and grandparents on the one hand, while supporting children and grandchildren on the other. They are generally isolated, poorly supported, unfunded, unorganized, and at risk. But, they are unable to avoid what they increasingly see as an ethical imperative, even if they must pay a significant price. And pay a price they do. Seventeen percent leave their jobs, twenty percent take anti-anxiety or anti-depressive medication, and 42 percent of those caring for a relative with dementia, in one study, were themselves clinically depressed.[6]

The second trend is health consumerism. It is difficult to fully appreciate that this movement only really began to take off in and around 1983, as part of the Civil Rights movement. People collectively woke up one day and confronted Health Emancipation. "These are our bodies," they said, "and we should be responsible for managing our own health decisions." To the great credit of physicians, nurses, and other caregivers in the United States and around the world, we agreed. What immediately ensued was two decades of health information empowerment with transfers of the scientific lexicon and the knowledge of basic organ function, the processes of chronic disease, and the beginnings of how to best prevent these diseases. Today 90 percent of physicians and patients in America agree the best patient is an educated patient.[7]

So in two short decades we have moved from emancipation to empowerment, and now find the movement morphing once again into active engagement. On the leading edge of this second wave of change are those third-generation women family caregivers I just referenced, who, confronted with managing the complexities and inefficiencies of the current system, have had enough, and are demanding that health care transform to better service their multigenerational needs. As they seize control, we are seeing increased focus on chronic disease management, palliative care, aging in place, and issues of death and dying. But we are also seeing our third-generation partners, as they reflect on their image in the mirror of parents and grandparents, examine their own and their children's and grandchildren's likely futures. The net effect is a growing emphasis on life-cycle planning and lifespan management.

In many ways, the people and people caring for the people are discovering this new approach in tandem in the public square. Consider osteoporosis. On first glance, it is a problem of the fourth and fifth generation. After all, there are over 1.5 million fragile fractures in elderly women in the United States each year. But, on second glance, studies show that in women age 50, 52 percent already have early bone loss and 20 percent have silent clinical osteoporosis. So perhaps this is a third-generation disease. But then there is the disturbing fact that by age 20, 98 percent of a woman's skeleton is formed. Now we're into the second generation. But then again, we have clearly established that fitness, nutrition, exercise, and avoiding smoking all contribute to skeletal formation in the first two decades of life.[8] And so it is with all chronic diseases. As we walk down the generational ladder, we arrive at preventive strategies and the need for advanced lifecycle planning. The 55-year-old woman caring for her mother with osteoporosis is not only trying to effectively support her mother's mobility and dignity, and alleviate her pain. She is also considering what she can do for herself, her daughter, and her granddaughter to avoid the same fate. The point to remember is that health consumerism has today become increasingly activist and focused on the concept of multigenerational health and prevention.

The third major trend is the evolution of the patient-physician relationship. Studies over the past nine years in the United States, United Kingdom, Germany, South Africa, Japan, and Canada have demonstrated that citizens in all of these countries value this relationship second only to family relationships. They see their relationship with their physicians as far more important than financial, spiritual, and co-worker relations. As consumers have evolved, so have their physicians. They have moved away from paternalism to partnerships, from individual to team approaches, and from clinical leadership to clinical, educational, and social leadership. Both patients and physicians define their relationship not in scientific but in social terms, as compassion, understanding, and partnership. The same is true for nurses, therapists, and the broad array of diverse caregivers.[9]

The fourth major trend has been the emergence of the Internet. For most, of course, the Internet represents a globally distributed information system with extraordinary reach and penetration, armed now, as well, with the capacity to encourage and facilitate personalized research. But for me, the most revolutionary element of the Internet is its capacity to ignore geographic boundaries that contain and define human populations. The Internet, if broadly accessible, has the potential power to eliminate geographic prejudices. For those who are disabled, elderly, poor, forgotten, and socially isolated, the Internet provides reason for hope, for it decreases our ability to isolate peoples and problems, whether local or global, and amplifies their voices. The Internet reveals the truth and places a glaring spotlight on inequities. So we are able to see in real time the juxtaposition of a member of the Masai tribe in Africa surviving on four liters of water per day in the shadow of the Los Angelean citizen consuming more than 500 liters of water per day. We are able to see and better understand that the developing world's exportation of infectious diseases—such as HIV/AIDS, SARS, and H5N1 bird flu—to the developed nations has been quickly returned in kind by the developed world's exportation of heavily marketed tobacco, poor nutrition, the weapons of war, and, today, war itself, which rapidly morphs into chronic disease and disability. So together, the Internet forces us to acknowledge that our global failures have created—for developing and developed world alike—a common reality: a shared dual burden of disease.[10]

On an economic and political scale, the Internet is equally transformational. Its combination with overnight delivery undermines geographically defined markets and market pricing. Markets represent a social agreement. For example, Canadian citizens accept somewhat decreased access to new health products and services in return for somewhat lower pricing, compared with their neighbors, for those entities. But with the Internet, each global citizen has the potential power to create his or her own market, cherry picking the best quality and most advantageous pricing from the comfort of home. More than this, most licensure and certification is geographically governed. Thus, in the United States, physicians, nurses, and pharmacists practice with the blessing of state bodies, in spite of the fact that Internet-based health commerce regularly crosses both state and national boundaries in today's virtual world.[11]

Finally, the Internet provides a single platform for the people and the people caring for the people to debate the pressing policy issues of the day. The Internet has the ability to accelerate consensus and to expand insight as events, exploding on different sides of the world, inform each other. It matters little in the end whether it's a tsunami or Hurricane Katrina. Bad policy is bad policy.

The fifth and final trend that bears mentioning is the emergence of non-governmental organizations, or NGOs. The first recorded NGO was the International Red Cross and Red Crescent movement, which sprang to life in Switzerland in 1863.[12] Nearly 40 years later, it formally arrived on U.S. soil.

For most of the following century, there was little growth in members or size of non-governmental associations. All of that began to change in the 1980s, for two critically important reasons. The first was the Internet, which resolved the nagging problem of limited resources that had plagued these fledgling issue-driven organizations. With the arrival of the Internet, NGO leaders quickly realized that they had been handed an incredibly efficient tool to solicit, organize, communicate, witness, advocate, and execute on a global scale. The second enabling force was media perception. As the 80s became the 90s, traditional broadcast and print media turned toward NGO leaders and away from government, business and academic leaders as credible sources and spokespeople for issue-oriented information and comment. Media credibility ratings of NGO leaders exceed 50 percent, while media credibility ratings of government and business leaders languish below 20 percent. The ability, then, of NGOs to execute off of a new media platform, while circling back to capture the power and impact of traditional media, created an explosive combination so that by the turn of the century, the number of NGOs had exceeded 20,000. This occurred as the waves of consumer-driven populism gained strength, reinforcing the strategic positioning of hard-hitting advocacy organizations over the more traditional, and some would say elitist and paternalistic, government, business, and educational institutions.[13]

So in a short 25 years, we have seen emerge the pressing demographics of aging with companion multigenerational complexity and the creation of the informal family caregiver movement; the birth of health consumerism and its evolution from emancipation to educational empowerment and now to active engagement; the transformation of the patient-physician relationship to support partnerships, team approaches, and joint decision-making; the emergence and massive expansion of the Internet, which refuses to play by the rules or pay homage to geography or traditional power bases; and finally, the explosive growth of a new type of leader, perfectly aligned with a populist public, who is more than prepared to answer the question, "What have you done for the people today?"

3.

Aging and Multi-Generational Complexity

I n his book *The Virtues of Aging*, former President Jimmy Carter said, "You are old when regrets take the place of dreams."[1] His title is especially fitting today, since aging is making real advances in quantity and quality of years.

Clearly, we have entered an era of new longevity. One need only look at the trend lines to see that the senior block is growing in leaps and bounds. There are now close to 200 million global citizens over the age of 65. This number is projected to increase to 678 million by the year 2030.[2] In 2000, there were some 35 million Americans over the age of 65. This number will more than double to 79 million by 2050.[2] And the oldest old, those over 85 years of age, are growing as well, from 4 million in 2000 to a projected 18 million in 2050.[3]

The numbers alone imply a fundamental shift in the American family. Nearly 50 percent of all current 60-year-olds have at least one parent alive. This means that the four-generation American family has arrived. By the year 2050, there will be an estimated 1 million Americans over the age of 100, making the five-generation American family commonplace.[3]

Even today, we can see the impact of these demographics on our day-to-day lives. Despite the fact that we've seen a 15 percent drop in the presence of chronic disability and institutionalization in our older population, largely as a result of improvements in medical care, technology, and lifestyle behavior, we still have a long way to go.[4]

One need not look far for evidence that American families are having trouble keeping up with changing demographics. Home care of dependent, frail seniors falls predominantly on third-generation women, who struggle to manage up and down the generation divide. Family and friends provide 80 percent of long-term care.[5] The inability to adequately address chronic disease ensures organ damage and disability. This cycle has created the "The Sandwich Generation," which finds itself squeezed between children and grandchildren on the right, and parents and grandparents on the left.

While clearly the demographics of aging seem overwhelming, reinforced by "boomers," who begin to hit 65 in 2011, there are forces deflecting the impact. In fact, poor health is not as prevalent in the elderly as we once thought. A full 75 percent of 65- to 74-year-olds consider themselves in good health, and 67 percent of those over 75 give themselves similar grades.[6]

Dr. Gene Cohen, while director of the Center of Aging, Health and Humanities at George Washington University, said, "The better health, higher level of education, and larger number of individuals with ample financial assets among today's older population—compared with earlier aging cohorts—speak to the greater collective role that those age 65 and older can play in assisting contemporary society."[7]

It's a race then: advancing age and traditional chronic, disease-instigated disability against advancing health and systems to support individual vitality and independence. Science and prevention must keep one step ahead of the demographic changes. A starting point is a clear understanding of the leading causes of death and disability in seniors.

The top five causes of mortality for those over 65 are heart disease, cancer, stroke, emphysema, and pneumonia. The top five sources of disability are arthritis, high blood pressure, heart disease, hearing impairments, and cataracts.[8]

The risk factors most likely to interfere with successful aging include smoking, alcohol abuse, depression, lack of exercise, and incontinence.[9,10,11] Addressing these behavioral issues can postpone the onset of disability by at least five years.[12]

Maintaining the functional capacity of aging Americans is critical to the long-term financing of health care. The direct health care costs for a chronically disabled senior are seven times greater than for a healthy senior.[12] The cost of care for a senior with dementia is 70 percent higher than a senior without mental impairment.[13] And none of this considers the indirect cost on family caregivers. A recent study of family caregivers of Alzheimer's patients found the average caregiver missed 23 days of work per year.[14]

So the challenge is clear: There must be a concerted effort on two fronts if the advance of health is to keep step with the advance of longevity. The first front is health mainte-nance. Currently, the average 75-year-old in America has three chronic conditions and takes 4.5 medications.[3] Early diagnosis, effective treatment, and healthy behaviors must continue to lower these numbers.

The second front is prevention. There's a great deal that can be done to better manage the changes and disabilities that are associated with aging. One simple example is hip fractures—mainly the result of poor supervision and unsafe environments for seniors—which are growing at an alarm-ing rate and projected to hit a half-million per year by 2050, with half of the injured never regaining independence.[3] Good management could positively impact those numbers.

PREVENTING ILLNESS, MAINTAINING HEALTH

We have clearly entered a new era of longevity in the United States and worldwide. This reality has political, social, eco-nomic, and health consequences that are fluid and not yet fully determined.

What we do know is that we will live longer and that four- and five-generation American families will be the norm.

We also know that, because of the arrival of the "boomers," beginning in 2011, the projected increase in numbers of seniors and their future lifespans in America over the next 50 years will be unprecedented.[6] The projected increase in years for men and even more so for women is extraordinary, and this is in addition to an already added 28 years of life expectancy for Americans over the past century.[15]

Absent effective preventive measures and improved health management, senior health care costs will financially cripple our health care system. Currently, Americans over 65 represent 13 percent of all hospital care, and 50 percent of all physician work hours.[4] But there are positive signs on the horizon. First, seniors' disability rates are declining in the United States. Since 1980 there has been a nearly 15 percent decrease in the prevalence of chronic disability and institutionalization among people 65 and older.[12] A drop in disability translates directly into cost savings since it is seven times more expensive to care for a disabled senior versus a healthy one.[3]

A second reason for optimism is that boomers are healthier than their parents. Earlier diagnosis and treatment of chronic diseases, behavioral changes in diet and exercise, and the health consumer empowerment movement have each played a role.[3] And the third sign of positive change is that both science and technology are progressing and contributing to a better understanding of diseases and the execution of methods to both diagnose and treat them.

If that is the good news, what are the concerns? One major concern is that our country is poorly prepared from a health-professional manpower standpoint to properly manage the complexity of aging. The average 75-year-old today has multiple chronic diseases and is on several medicines, yet fewer than one percent of all physicians, nurses, pharmacists, and physical therapists have had advanced geriatric training.[4] How does this disconnect play out? Let's take just one case in point, the under-diagnosis of depression in the elderly—an easy miss if you've not been alerted by your training to look for it, and if you've been raised in the age of, "Mom's slowing down is just part of her getting old."

Depression is often misdiagnosed as cognitive impairment, in spite of the fact that there are many good reasons to be depressed: retirement, widowhood, bereavement, and isolation.[4] But the cause of depression can be much more subtle. For example, having a hearing impairment is frequently associated with depression. More aggressive approaches to hearing loss would be very beneficial. Hearing loss affects quality of life and interpersonal relationships, and is a significant safety issue.[16] And if other diseases cause depression in the elderly, the reverse is true as well. Depression increases the risk of disability from all other causes in the elderly by 67 percent.[16] Training in geriatrics sensitizes clinicians to these various interactions.

A second concern is treatment strategies. Where should we begin? A logical starting point is with cognitive impairment. There are some four million American seniors currently suffering from Alzheimer's disease and dementia, with numbers expected to reach 14 million by 2040. The numbers increase with age. While 2 percent may have the disease at age 65, 16 percent are affected by 85.[17] The costs are staggering, estimated in 2000 at $100 billion per year, making it the third most expensive disease in the United States.[18] Nearly 50 percent of all nursing home patients are cognitively impaired.[4] The scientific focus on neurodegenerative diseases in both public and private sectors is enormous, and reflects both the seriousness of the problem and the potential positive impact that would accompany a solution.

Where else is there significant paydirt? Incontinence affects 13 million Americans, including half of all nursing patients, at a cost of nearly $12 billion per year.[19] Experts suggest that we also target other conditions that lead to institutionalization. Major activity limitations are a common cause of nursing home admissions. The most common cause is arthritis, affecting 50 percent of people over 65, and an estimated 60 million people by 2020.[20] Hip fractures are a second source of immobility, projected to occur 420,000 times in the year 2020, nearly all fall-related, resulting in a loss of independence in nearly 30 percent of those affected. Fully 80 percent occur in women, who are at special risk because of osteoporosis.[4]

In addition to the obvious benefits of medical treatment and the creation of safe environments, the expansion of exercise and muscle strengthening could make a real difference in the incidence of falls and fractures. At present, even minimal exercise is totally absent in one-third of those over 65, and weight training is nearly nonexistent.[21]

Finally, a focus on medications, their interactions, assistance in their accurate and regular administration, and regular evaluation would lead to further improvement.

Dollars spent on both geriatric training and the prevention of those conditions most likely to cause disability and institutionalization are an extraordinarily wise investment. Adding a single month of independence and health to America's senior population would save $5 billion. A 10 percent decrease in hospitalization and institutionalization would accrue $50 billion in savings per year.[3]

But is good health simply delaying the inevitable, a long and expensive deterioration occurring later in life? Surprisingly, no. Studies of centenarians have shown that their decades of relative good health are followed by a highly compressed period of compromised health at the end of life.[22]

NEW ENVIRONMENTS FOR MATURE LIVING

Donna Shalala, secretary of Health and Human Services at the turn of the 20th century, said: "We want life not only to be long, but good. This will be one of the central challenges of the 21st Century: to make dignity and comfort for the elderly as much a part of our national consciousness as education and safety are for our children."[23]

We are in a scientific and social service race against the very real challenges of aging demographics. This requires a two-pronged strategy. The first arm is enlightened prevention and health maintenance, intended to help elders maintain vitality and independence for as long as possible by aggressively addressing those conditions that lead to disability and institutionalization.

The second arm, which is complementary to the first, is the creation of new environments that actively manage the changes and disabilities that come with advanced age. Long-term care is part of the natural fabric of life. It is fundamentally different than acute care in that it integrates health services and supports for daily living. The explosive growth of the long-term care industry simply reflects the numbers, with a projected doubling of the over-65s and tripling of the over-85s in the next 50 years.[24,25] During this period, the number of people requiring long-term care is projected to grow from less than 10 million to 24 million.[26] But one should not confuse our future vision of long-term care with older images of restrictive nursing homes.

Even with excellent health maintenance and prevention, most of us will need to confront the issue of long-term care. Fully 43 percent of those over 65 will require some long-term care services in their lifetime, including 52 percent of all women and 33 percent of all men.[27] What's more, 51 percent of all Americans believe that it is likely that in their lifetime they will be responsible for the care of an elderly family member.[28]

What is it that causes individuals to require this support? The need for long-term care is measured by the limitation in capacity to perform certain basic functions or activities called "Activities of Daily Living," or ADLs. ADLs include bathing, dressing, getting in and out of bed, eating, toileting, and moving about. There are other activities, called "Instrumental Activities of Daily Living," or IADLs, such as getting out, driving, preparing meals, shopping, maintaining a home, using a phone, managing finances, and taking medications, which are critical and require help if absent, though not on the level of absent ADLs.

About 97 percent of nursing home patients have ADL limitations.[26] By age 85, the need for help is not at all unusual. Some 35 percent need assistance with walking, 31 percent with bathing, 22 percent with getting in and out of bed, 17 percent with dressing, 14 percent with toileting, and 4 percent with eating.

Most of those requiring long-term care prefer to "age in place," in their own home and community, in familiar settings. And most do just that. In fact, the use of nursing homes is declining in all categories of aging, with numbers of nursing home patients over 85 declining by nearly 10 percent between 1985 and 1995.[29] Instead, what we see is nearly 90 percent of seniors living in their own homes, independently or with informal care that's almost always provided by family or close friends. This compares with 4.5 percent who are living at home with professional care and 4.6 percent residing in nursing homes.[30]

The primary challenge for providing long-term care support for fourth and fifth generation Americans is falling predominantly on third generation female family members. As Jim Firman, president of the National Council on Aging has noted, "We mistakenly define long-term care problems as medical concerns rather than disability concerns. The care needs of most frail older people are primarily supportive: for example, help them move from here to there, help them eat and dress, and help them keep track of their medicine."[31]

If family members provide the muscle of home care, they also provide a significant portion of the dollars. For 40 percent of Americans, long-term care is the most costly purchase ever made.[32] More than 32 percent of the total costs of long-term care in 1999 came directly from patients, while the government shouldered approximately 56 percent of the bill—38 percent in Medicaid and 18 percent in Medicare. Only 5.5 percent was covered by private insurance.[33]

As family members critically assess the financial consequences of these difficult decisions, costs are being assigned to each option. The ability to live independently at home is less expensive than institutionalization. But, as Gail Hunt, executive director of The National Alliance for Caregiving, says, "There's a reason for that. The quality of life at home is better, yes, but only the federal government saves money. And that's because family caregivers are the unpaid extensions of the health care system." In 1992 it was roughly five times more expensive to be elderly and dependent in a nursing home versus independent in one's own home.[34] The nursing home charge then averaged $29,000 per year. Today, the cost exceeds $60,000 per year.[34,35]

The race against the aging juggernaut, then, is about science, about independence, and about "aging in place." Long-term care is rapidly evolving with a primary focus on dignity, personal autonomy, and support for caregivers.

What are the major trends in long-term care? First, less institutionalized care. Nursing homes are being reserved for the most severely impaired. Second, more reliance on home care and community-based alternatives. Day care options, blended services, "assisted living," and care for the caregiver programs all signal a shift in emphasis that presages a shift in finances. Third, these environments will feature more choices, greater use of supportive new life-assist technologies, a greater emphasis on prevention, and the opportunity for shared learning and community-based strategic planning.

If one were to plan, what might emerge as the best environment for mature living? It would be a place that supports dignity and privacy, a place that balances personal autonomy with safety, a place that leverages technology to enhance personal security and safety, a place that provides stimulation and social interaction, and a place that ensures easy access to affordable services.

There is a great deal of work to be done to get ahead of the aging curve. But we should be optimistic for two reasons.

The solution relies on the goodness of America's individuals, families, and communities on the one hand, and on the power of innovation imbedded in America's scientific and medical enterprise on the other.

4.

Lifespan Management and the Leadership of Women

In 1996, shortly before he died, the great Cardinal Bernadine of Chicago addressed an annual meeting of the American Medical Association and said; "There are four words in the English language that have common English roots. They are heal, health, whole, and holy. I tell you this because to heal in a modern world you must provide health. And for there to be health, you must keep the individual, the family, the community, and society whole. And if you can do all that, well that is a holy thing."

What we have come to understand since Cardinal Bernadine uttered those words is that it is impossible to move this vision without the leadership of women who are both healthy and enlightened and prepared to champion individual and family health. In the 21st Century, we realize that gender has a direct effect on health and well-being. We have a growing appreciation that women's health is not only affected by reproduction, but also by unique biological systems and complex social and economic roles.

What we see emerging is not only an expansion of knowledge and empowerment, but also an increasing effort to organize and prioritize needs in women's health. Key areas of focus now include the expansion of numbers of women in clinical trials, a concentration on accessible health care services available to women and their families, an expansion of informational empowerment, and an emphasis on lifespan management.

If there are challenges in prioritizing resources around women's health, those challenges are made all the more complex by major shifts presently occurring in the health care industry. First, we see a continued movement away from reactive treatment toward proactive prevention. Second, we are moving away from an organ-centric approach with a single focus on reproductive capabilities toward a broader, gender-based construct. And third, we are looking toward systems of insurance that are key to ensuring early access to lifelong continuums of care.

To effectively provide women with appropriate health care services, an awareness of lifespan is critical. Dr. Donna Dean of the National Institutes of Health recently said, "I do not know if the public truly understands that prevention needs to start very early in a woman's life. Osteoporosis is a good example. It is really a disease for which preventative steps need to start in childhood. If we started good health care practices at that age, we probably would not have as big a problem at the other end of the age spectrum."[1]

If a woman's lifespan is uniquely integrated, it is also uniquely segmented, with critical health needs and challenges at each stage. In the adolescent years, self-esteem is a critical health determinant. A study of 4,000 girls age 14 to 18 conducted by Seventeen magazine revealed that 50 percent would consider cosmetic surgery, 50 percent were dissatisfied with their weight and shape, and 65 percent were tired, stressed, and burned-out.[2] By age 15, girls were twice as likely as boys to experience a major depressive episode, a gender gap that is sustained through age 50.[3] Indeed, women attempt suicide two to three times as often as men.[4] And nearly 4 percent of young women in this study suffered from a significant eating disorder.[5] In spite of those very real risks, teenage girls often have limited contact with physicians, falling between the cracks of pediatric and reproductive care. Leading health concerns among women 25 to 44 shift to childbearing and infertility. In the 21st Century, women are bearing children later in life and experiencing a higher incidence of infertility. In 1996, the percentage of childless women age 20 to 24 was 65 percent, age 25 to 29, 44 percent, and age 30 to 34, 26 percent.[6] A study reported in 2002 found that 33 percent of professional women age 28 to 55 were childless, while only 14 percent wished to be child-free.[7] More than 6 million Americans suffer from infertility, half of them women.[8]

The focus on reproduction in women age 25 to 44 tends to overshadow other health concerns, including important causes of death and disability such as cancer, accidents and violence, heart disease and HIV/AIDS.[6] The incidence of HIV among American women, for example, is on the rise and was the fifth leading cause of death among Caucasian women and the leading cause of death among African-American women as we entered the new millenium.[9] The reproductive years provide greater contact with the health care system and, potentially, a unique opportunity to aggressively address these non-reproductive health care risks.

During the middle years, women encounter expanded responsibilities, menopause, and a number of serious health issues. Women spend more than one-third of their lives in the post-reproductive menopausal years. In the United States, the average age of menopausal onset is 51.[10] In addition to managing the physical and emotional symptoms of menopause, vigilance is required on a number of health fronts. One-third of 45- to 64-year-olds, and 55 percent of women over 65, experience arthritis. More than 50 percent will experience osteoporosis-related fractures during their lifetimes. Approximately 11 percent of 45- to 64-year-olds have heart disease, with one-third over 65 affected. And those over 50 are responsible for 77 percent of the new cases of breast cancer and 70 percent of the new cases of cervical cancer.[11,12,13,14,15] In all of these situations, prevention, early diagnosis, and effective treatment are life-enhancing and life-saving.

But women of this age group often find little time to care for themselves. Responsibilities for others—parents, grandparents, spouses, children, and grandchildren—too often mean that a middle-aged woman's own health comes last. There are more than 25 million family caregivers in the United States, with rates highest among women 45 to 64.[16] Women who are caregivers are more likely to have health problems, with 54 percent having one or more chronic conditions compared with 41 percent of non-caregivers, and 51 percent with high depressive symptoms compared with 38 percent of the control population.[17]

As the years advance, older women carry a disproportionate burden of chronic diseases, in part because they have longer lifespans than men.[18] Fully 22 percent of U.S. women will be over 65 by 2030.[19] In women 65 to 74, cancer is the leading cause of death, while heart disease dominates in those over 75.[6] As important, there is the ever-present risk of disability. Today, 23 million American women have osteoporosis.[20]

DISEASES AND RISK FACTORS

In women's health, knowledge alone does not equal power. Knowledge, combined with the willingness and ability to act on that knowledge, equals power. Dr. Andrea Pennington, the medical director for DiscoveryHealth.com, recently observed, "We are currently in a 'need-to-know' era in terms of health information. But tomorrow will bring the start of a 'need-to-act' era. Women need actionable instructions."

Relevant information is key. We know that a woman's health span is uniquely integrated across a lifetime, and uniquely segregated, with each phase of life containing its own distinct health concerns. That said, there are major risks and key diseases that represent a general threat across a woman's entire life spectrum.

The risk of cardiovascular disease is a major one that women "need to know" about and "act on." What are the risk factors for cardiovascular disease? First, smoking, which causes one-and-a-half times more deaths from heart disease than from lung cancer.[21] Smokers are two to six times more likely than non-smokers to suffer a heart attack.[21] Second, physical inactivity: 60 percent of women fail to meet moderate exercise requirements, and 25 percent do not exercise at all.[22] Third, nutrition: approximately one-third of American women are obese, and one-fourth have high cholesterol levels.[21,23] Fourth, high blood pressure: 52 percent of women over 45 have elevated blood pressure.[23] And finally, diabetes represents a more significant risk to women than men. Women with diabetes are nearly twice as likely as men to suffer from heart disease.[23]

The additive effect of those risk factors creates a startling reality for women. In 1997, more than 500,000 women in the United States died of heart disease, compared to 450,000 men. Smoking and taking oral contraceptives after age 35 is an especially deadly combination. Currently, it is estimated that more than 20 percent of all U.S. women have cardiovascular disease. When women have heart attacks, they are more likely than men to die within a year—42 percent compared to 24 percent. And African-American women's risk of a cardiovascular-related death exceeds that of white women by nearly 15 percent.[24]

A second major concern is cancer. While breast cancer remains the most common cancer among women, each year lung cancer is responsible for more women's deaths.[25,26] In fact, lung cancer deaths among men are dropping, even as rates among women rise.[25] In 1998, 22 percent of surveyed women smoked. Those numbers are increasing.[27] In 2000, 30 percent of high school senior girls smoked. Three million U.S. women have died from smoking-related causes since 1980, and it's estimated that more than 50 percent of those cancers were preventable.[27]

Depression is a third major threat to women across their entire lifecycle. The incidence of depression in women is twice that seen in men, affecting 12 percent versus 6 percent.[28] Teenage girls are especially vulnerable as they adjust to physical and hormonal changes, emerging sexuality, and parental control issues. These all translate to higher rates of depression, anxiety, eating disorders, and disruptive behaviors.[29] As women enter young adulthood, fluctuations in reproductive hormones affect levels of neurotransmitters and their circadian rhythms.[30] Adult women are also exposed to a wider array of adverse life events associated with depression, the most recent addition being adult caregiving responsibilities. Finally, women frequently outlive their husbands. About 800,000 women per year are widowed and left to sort through loneliness, feelings of abandonment, and an array of complex management responsibilities and choices.[29]

A fourth major issue, often overlooked or swept under the rug, is violence and abuse. Studies show that 40 percent of all U.S. women have been subjected to violence.[17] Some 12 million women are victims of rape: 700,000 in a 12-month period, with 60 percent occurring before the age of 18, and 84 percent never being reported to the police.[31] Additionally, 31 percent of all women experience domestic violence. This is not simply confined to the poor. While one-half of all women with annual incomes less than $16,000 are affected by domestic violence, so too are one-third of those with incomes over $50,000.[17] Increasingly, the long-term connection between violence and poor health is being established. At least part of the story is tied to a higher incidence of secondary risk factors. Abused women are twice as likely to smoke as those not abused. They are also 40 percent more likely to drink and 34 percent more likely to be depressed.

The fifth major issue is HIV/AIDS and STDs among teenage girls and young women.[32] As we crossed into the new century, there were three million cases of chlamydia annually, 45 million cases of genital herpes, and 20 million cases of Human Papilloma Virus in women. While 9 percent were infected in 1989, by 1997, 15 percent were infected. In 2002, the number stood at 25 percent. Between 1989 and 1998, the incidence of HIV/AIDS among women age 13 to 19 increased 18 times. Minority women carried most of that burden. While African-American and Hispanic-American women comprise 23 percent of America's female population, they represent 76 percent of all U.S. women infected with HIV/AIDS.[9,33]

There is, then, a "need-to-act" as well as a "need-to-know." What are the impediments to acting on our current knowledge of women's health?

OVERCOMING OBSTACLES

In the first two parts of this chapter we have examined the unique challenges encountered in women's health care. On the one hand, those challenges are tied to lifespans, which possess a high level of age-span segmentation. For example, the distinct challenges and risk factors in adolescence, compared with the very different health concerns of a woman in the middle years. On the other hand, a woman's health often involves a high level of integration. For example, the destructive seeds of elder osteoporosis are planted by poor nutrition habits set at an early age. We have also examined the major risk factors and disease entities that challenge women at different stages in their lives.

Now let's focus on the obstacles that must be overcome to advance women's health in the 21st Century. Being healthy means different things to different women. The obstacles to health, therefore, are a function of the differing expectations of women. Nancy Fugate Woods, dean of the School of Nursing at the University of Washington, explored this issue in a study of 500 Seattle women. Those women, she noted, "said that being free of disease was just one part of good health. Many spoke about how being healthy meant being able to deal with the stresses and strains that were part of their daily lives, being able to perform optimally at whatever their roles were in society, whether that was going to work, taking care of their kids, or being responsible for caregiving.

And then there were some women who talked about health in a different way, as achieving a high level of wellness, really having a sense of feeling good."[34]

A primary and fundamental obstacle to the advancement of women's health is the fragmented nature of health care itself. Approximately 37 percent of all adult women routinely see two different doctors for their health care. Communication between those caregivers is in no way ensured.[35] As Dr. Carol Weisman of the University of Michigan School of Public Health observes, "Women see multiple providers for primary care: OB-GYNs, family practitioners, general internists, advanced practice nurses, and others." In many communities, different services are located in different places. Scheduling can be a problem too. The burden on women to access and coordinate their care is also likely to worsen as women age and develop multiple conditions.[1]

The business of being a healthy 21st Century woman takes a lot of work, and that work gets imposed on an already overworked and aging population. Dr. Evelyn Murphy, head of Women's Studies at Brandeis University, says, "Until we learn to match services with time constraints of the working woman, we cannot expect her to take the most simple precautionary measures, much less the more time-consuming ones, because it jeopardizes her job. Her job may already be in jeopardy if she is taking personal time off due to illness. Then she is nervous as well as ill. And of course, anxiety cannot be good for her health."[1]

A study commissioned by Women's Policy, Inc., and published in 2000, revealed that at best we were only two-thirds of the way to good, basic preventive health care for women. Only 61 percent of women over 50 had undergone a complete physical exam in the past year, 64 percent a pap smear, 66 percent a breast exam; 55 percent a blood cholesterol test, and 69 percent a mammogram.

If the absence of time is a serious obstacle, the absence of money compounds the problem. Poverty is a significant determinant of poor health in women. Dr. Robert Rebar of the American Society for Reproductive Medicine states, "I honestly think that when it comes to providing health care for poor women, we did a better job 25 years ago than we do today."[1] Issues of poverty impact women of all ages. Poor women have higher levels of unintended and unattended pregnancies. They have higher levels of chronic diseases and disability. They have higher levels of depression and anxiety. More women are poorer than men, and time off for diagnosis and treatment is less often an option for poor women. And if time off is not an option when they are young, then the same is often true when they get old.[17]

Add to time and money the unique logistical demands of managing up and down the four- and five-generation American divide. Women now care for parents and grandparents as they tend to children and grandchildren. There are some 25 million informal family caregivers at work in the United States.[17] Of those, 70 percent are women 45 to 64. One-fifth of women caregivers change their work status to manage family responsibilities: 7 percent go part-time, 6.4 percent quit their jobs altogether, and 11 percent take a leave of absence.[36] This is not the only sacrifice they make. One-quarter subsequently describe their own health as fair or poor. And their perception of poor health is "on the mark" according to a recent study of interleukin six levels in caregivers. This chemical marker of stress and aging increased six times faster in caregivers of family members with dementia than in a non-caregiving matched cohort.[17]

So women's health is very much a woman's issue. But success in defining and executing strategies to advance the health of America's women—the primary caregivers, health coordinators, and wellness motivators of America's increasingly complex and aging and home-based family—will realize unparalleled benefits, not only to women, but to families, communities, and our society overall.

5.

A Focus on the Home

Some 40 years ago, I recall visiting General Electric's "Carousel of Progress" at the World's Fair in New York with my girlfriend (now my wife). The attraction, now housed at Disney World in Florida, documented the changes in the technology and social structure of the American home over five or six decades, ultimately creating a vision of the future, a case for progress. I think the time has come to build something similar for health care. This "Carousel of Health" would provide a vision of the past, present, and future for something far more important than refrigerators and toasters—our nation's health. At the core of this carousel would be a vision that's just within our reach—something that will change health care as we now know it. I'm talking about the concept of home-centered health, in which technology, advanced information systems, and a new, more team-oriented medical approach would make it possible for individuals to reconnect with each other and for more health care to take place in the home than we ever imagined possible.

Today, voices are rising once again in the name of health care reform. The various power bases remain much as they were in 1980—locked in position, facing year-to-year battles for funding support from fixed public and private sources. While they have not changed, the health care world certainly has. We are now immersed in a full-blown health consumer empowerment movement in response to aging demograph-ics, a caregiver revolution, advances in information technol-ogy, debates over risks and benefits of various treatments and therapies, and an outpatient office-based delivery system that lacks time and space to advance prevention and wellness.

In the middle of all this noise, quietly below the radar screen, health care is preparing to restructure itself from the inside out through a "parallel build-out." At the end of this silent evolution, we will have a home-centered health care system that will radically realign the current players and power bases. The new system will tilt rewards to those who play prevention, and play it well.[1]

At the center of this home-centered health scenario will be the American family—aging in place, now routinely four and five generations deep, rather than just three. Family caregiv-ers, currently present in 25 percent of American families, are providing most of the care for parents and grandparents.[2] In the next decade, they will embrace the designated role of home health manager and apply their skills up and down the generational divide as designated members of physicians' health care teams.[3]

Those teams will carry out both educational and clinical missions. The educational support teams will be coordi-nated with physicians' active support, primarily by nurse educators connected 24/7 to virtual networks of family-based home health managers. Through this network, home health managers will receive targeted education, behavioral modification strategies, and financial rewards in the form of reduced insurance premiums for achieving superior out-comes for family members. Physicians, as well, will be tied to performance and fairly reimbursed for team management responsibilities.[4]

The home itself will look quite different—it will generally be more stable, productive, and controlled. Technology will play a dual role. Originally directed at seniors with cognitive decline, cancer, and cardiovascular disease who wanted to age in place, it will now be harnessed to advance the health of all ages.[5] The infrastructure for maintaining home-based wellness will include wireless sensors that track movement of people and objects in-home; intelligent software that will analyze data and provide appropriate behavioral clues and guidance; friendly, communicative interfaces through a wide range of devices, such as wristwatches, telephones, and televisions; and Internet and wireless connectivity with the rest of the health care team.[6]

This could become our reality, but the pieces must fall into place. According to David Tennenhouse, former vice president and director of Intel Research, "The real challenge for research now is to explore the implications and issues associated with having hundreds of networked computers per person. These networked computers will work together to learn our habits and patterns and be proactive in providing us with the information and services we need for a healthier, safer, more productive, and enjoyable life."[5]

In the near future, such systems could adjust behavior in physical fitness, nutrition, social activity, and cognitive engagement. They could assist seniors with incontinence, in regular toileting, and ensure better adherence to medication regimens. They could provide early diagnostics, streaming data daily to the physician-directed, nurse-led educational team, and adjust daily treatment regimens, support disease avoidance, and substantially decrease the need for on-site office visits or hospitalization.[5]

Intel is not alone in this vision. Massachusetts Institute of Technology, the University of Michigan, the University of Virginia, and the University of Rochester are just a few of the academic institutions actively engaged.[7,8,9,10] So are General Electric, NASA, the Disney spin-off i.d.e.a.s., Best Buy, and Philips, which all see home health technology as a major growth market.[11,12,13,14,15] Add to these, new health units at Google, Microsoft, and Revolution Health. They are all betting that the technology, privacy, and usability barriers can be overcome, and that once health consumers are at financial risk, the logic of prevention will prevail, and a tipping point will have been reached.

Why might they be right? First, there is inadequate funding, time, and space to manage an aging, actively disease-ridden population. Second, education, behavioral modification, and preventive screening must be home-based to be successful. Third, the complexity of a four- and five-generation family becomes rapidly unmanageable in the absence of active health planning and the deliberate transfer of learnings down the generational ladder. Fourth, success in managing home-based health prevention saves time and money, in the short and long term. Fifth, most people don't want to go to a hospital unless they absolutely have to.

Beyond all this, much of our future home-based health workforce is already in place—highly stressed, yet ready, willing, and able. I'm talking about the nation's informal caregivers, present in a quarter of all homes, 34 million strong. Seventy percent of these informal caregivers are women, age 45 to 64 years.[16,17] Ignore for the moment that 20 percent of them have been forced to sacrifice their work status to manage the complexity of caregiving and that nearly half of those managing elder dementia have symptoms of depression from the isolation and constant work load. Sadly, it's clear that what our family caregivers have learned has been hard fought and accomplished with very little help from the system.[18,19]

Now, let us admit these weaknesses and injustices, and recognize that a change in incentives, infrastructure, and goal-directed organization could increase job satisfaction and success for these dedicated workers. You might be wondering, "Who are these caregivers, and what qualifies them to be home health managers?"

A recent survey of 1,005 women, conducted by the National Women's Health Resource Center, begins to answer these questions.[20] Seventy-one percent of the women surveyed said they make health care decisions such as selecting a health care professional and choosing when to go to the physician for their family. According to Amy Niles, the group's president and chief executive officer, "Our study found that caring for the health of others is perceived to have a major positive impact on women's physical and mental health. Given these findings, it is not surprising that women choose to take on the role of health manager for their family, making the bulk of health care-related decisions."

When women in the study were asked to identify areas that are "very important" to them, 96 percent chose "having a healthy family"; 95 percent chose "being healthy"; and 90 percent said "being close to family." This is all the more remarkable when compared with some of the other results. Only 72 percent of the women said "being financially secure" was "very important"; 66 percent said "having close friends"; and 65 percent said "having a job you enjoy." Only 40 percent said "having enough free time" was "very important" to them.

Women are not only committed to their families' health, they are good at handling and understanding it. Many are consistently ahead of the curve. Fifty-five percent of women are aware that heart disease is the major killer of women; two-thirds are very familiar with their family's medical history; and 95 percent are knowledgeable about diagnosis and treatment of diseases their parents have suffered. It's clear that women are also familiar with and support screening guidelines such as Pap smears, teeth cleanings, and cholesterol tests. More than 90 percent have seen their physicians and other care professionals in the past year. Seventy-four percent are most likely to get their information on health issues from their health care professional, and 60 percent have used the Internet for information research.[20]

According to the results of the National Women's Health Resource Center survey, women's views of health are multidimensional and integrated, emphasizing body, mind, and spirit. When asked in the study to identify what "being healthy" means, "having a healthy family" ranked Number 1, followed by spiritual well-being, being happy, being physically active, not having chronic disease, and not being overweight. As for issues women consider contributors to unhealthiness, stress, lack of exercise, poor nutrition, and low income all scored high.[20]

Let me suggest for the moment that this workforce will expand as boomers age, and that some men of like mind will join. If we were to move from an informal to a formal home health workforce, what might be done to strengthen the home health managers' performance, longevity, and retention? First, have physicians include these managers as part of their health care team. Second, organize, on the local practice level, physician-led, nurse-directed "virtual teams" of home health managers to provide information and address isolation. Third, advocate for health insurance reform to reward home health managers for success in managing their multigenerational family's wellness and prevention. Fourth, support smart technology development to outfit homes for efficiency, connectivity, safety, education, and behavioral modification. Fifth, experiment with best practices that save time, lower stress, and build efficient, reliable care processes.

A home-centered health care system, where information begins at home, connects to physicians and care teams, and circles back home, seems impossible only because the pieces of our system, built long ago for vertical disease intervention, are locked in place by historic silos and outdated business plans. But we're now moving toward a horizontal model of health care, one that flattens the old silos, rearranges and reconstructs the pieces, and connects all the players together in a much more logical way.

As we enter this new millennium, we are experiencing a shifting health care value proposition. Americans are attempting to move from reactive intervention to proactive prevention, and this changes the playing field for everyone—hospitals, doctors' offices, health insurers, and pharmaceutical and medical device companies alike. It implies healthy behaviors, early diagnosis, regular screenings, knowing your numbers, effective long-term treatments with excellent adherence, and a personalized, information- and relationship-rich support system that is equitable and just. It suggests that to be valued in our future health care system, each player, in addition to his or her traditional unique contributions, will also need to be engaged in educational and behavioral modification to claim insider status.[16,21,22]

With these in mind, the health care "Carousel of Progress" has been created. Now, we're circling counter-clockwise and the last set appears. Ten realities have been skillfully integrated into this calm and well-organized vision of a healthy home:

1. A home health manager, previously the informal family caregiver, has been designated for each extended family.

2. Health insurance covers nearly all Americans, and a medical information highway has been constructed primarily around the patient, with caregivers integrated in, rather than the other way around.

3. The majority of prevention, behavioral modification, monitoring, and treatment of chronic diseases now takes place at home.

4. Physician-led, nurse-directed virtual health networks of home health managers provide a community-based, 24/7, educational and emotional support team.

5. Health care insurance premiums for families have just gone down due to expert performance of the home health manager, as reflected in outcome measures of family members.

6. Basic diagnostics, including blood work, imaging, vital signs, and therapeutics are performed automatically or by the home health manager

and transmitted electronically to the physician-led, nurse-directed educational network, which provides feedback, coaching, and treatment options as necessary.

7. Sophisticated behavioral modification tools, age-adjusted for each generation, are present and utilized, funded in part by diagnostic and therapeutic companies who have benefited from expansion of insurance coverage and health markets as early diagnosis, prevention, and lifespan health planning have, in concert with partners from the technology, entertainment, and financial sectors, taken hold.

8. Physician office capacity has grown, as most care does not require a visit. Physician reimbursement has increased in acknowledgement of their roles in managing clinical and educational teams and multigenerational complexity. Nursing school enrollment is up as the critical role as educational director of home health manager networks has become a major magnet for the profession.

9. Family nutrition is carefully planned and executed; activity levels of all five generations are up; weight is down; cognition is up; mental and physical well-being are also up.

10. Hospitals continue to right size—they're more specialized and safer, with better outcomes. And scientific advances have allowed early diagnosis and more effective treatment, making the need for hospitalization increasingly rare.

Is this all a far-fetched scenario? Not really. Many of these elements are well within the reach of an integrated and progressive vision for tomorrow's health. What is missing is our willingness to concentrate and focus on homes as the cornerstone of a new preventive health care system.

6.
Evolution of the Patient-Physician Relationship

The patient-physician relationship is at the epicenter of stable, civil, relationship-based societies. A national study, conducted in 1997, found that 90 percent of patients and physicians defined the relationship as having three elements: compassion, understanding, and partnership.[1] While science, technology, and professional competency were viewed as important in ensuring a successful relationship, they were separate from the very human emotions that bind patients to physicians—and physicians to patients.

On a broader scale, this relationship is clearly in the "middle of the mix." Both patients and physicians have important spheres of influence that they bring to the dance. And these spheres move within the orbit of a wide array of consumer, media, medical, regulatory, political, and research organizations.[2]

In 2002, studies in six countries on four continents revealed that the citizens of all countries viewed the patient-physician relationship as second in importance only to family relationships.[3] In the United States, the patient-physician relationship scored significantly higher than spiritual, financial, and co-worker relationships. This finding was repeated in the United Kingdom, Canada, Germany, South Africa, and

Japan. These high levels of confidence may, in part, reflect the fact that, in all countries studied, strong majorities believe that physicians place the patient's interests above anything else, and exhibit high levels of trust in their physicians to manage private patient data and information correctly.

While the relationship is highly valued, it is certainly not static. In all countries studied, the relationship is rapidly evolving. Authoritarian, paternalistic relationships—where "doctor says" and "patient does"—are now in the minority. They have been replaced by mutual partnerships with 50/50 decision-making, and advisor relationships where the physician serves as a resource and guide, but patients take responsibility for decisions.[3]

What's next? Patients worldwide state that the relationship will move further away from paternalism, to fully embrace one-on-one mutual partnerships, and expect to see continued movement toward service-oriented physician teams. These teams will not only deliver traditional clinical care—for example, with a coordinated group of medical professionals caring for a diabetic patient—but will also include a parallel educational team to support patient empowerment. The patient in this case would have the benefit of access to a wide array of professionals. In addition to the primary care physician, the patient would expect coordinated access to specialists as needed, nurse educators, nutritionists, physical therapists, mental health professionals, health librarians, web managers, self-help teams, consumer advocates, and others.

Studies show that patients are realistic and don't expect their physicians to do the educating themselves. But they do expect the physicians to provide oversight to the educational team, to validate their expertise, and to ensure that information is up-to-date and accurate. As educational support is growing, so too is patient confidence in self-management. Between 63 percent and 76 percent of patients in all countries studied, except Japan, are completely or very confident in managing their own health. And in Japan, 57 percent are somewhat confident, moving en masse toward health consumer empowerment.[3]

Empowerment is clearly a function of educational support. While physicians are the patient's primary source of information, this is only one factor in a formula for behavioral change. Physicians are also the most trusted source of information, and the professionals whose recommendations patients are most likely to follow. In all countries studied, the physicians' role in moving patients toward more active self-management is highly noted.[3]

In the United States alone, hundreds of thousands of times each day, on a grassroots level, these very private and highly charged relationships are engaged. The cost to society is not insignificant. But what is the true value? Certainly, the relationships deliver, to a significant portion of society, "nuts and bolts health care"—though irregularly and with a fragile and imperfect safety net. This includes diagnosis, treatment, and follow-up care, with greater emphasis still being placed on reactive intervention rather than on thoughtful prevention.

But this service alone hardly explains the high valuation of physicians. The true value, social science studies reveal, extends well beyond "nuts and bolts." The patient-physician relationship delivers three other important products each and every day.[4] First, it processes the populace's very private fears and worries, channeling most to a positive outcome. In so doing, it effectively vents societal anxiety that might otherwise accumulate to destabilizing effect. Second, in individualizing care within the context of family, community, and culture, the relationship quietly reinforces and affirms the value of individual connectivity to other cornerstone values and to contact points in society. Third, the relationship quietly and effectively instills hope and confidence in the future, which translates into a willingness to invest money, talent, and ideas that shape a society's future and the willingness to assume risk today in pursuit of goal tomorrow.

If the relationship is as highly valued, and the investment

made by most countries so significant, why is health care policy so often a source of controversy? Or, stated another way, why is all the money that's expended on health care not viewed as delivering sufficient value?

UNLOCKING THE VALUE

In the same study noted above, large majorities of physicians in all countries agreed with the statement: "The medical system in your country sometimes interferes with your ability to put your patient's interests above everything else." This conflict, felt by physicians, is not as visible to patients, who in large majorities, in the same study, agree strongly or somewhat that "the doctor puts my interests above everything else."[2]

What is the source of this fundamental disconnect between health care system design and its anchoring relationship? The problem in the United States can be traced to two factors: First, a fundamentally flawed understanding of the true value proposition in health care; and second, a lack of understanding of what defines the patient-physician relationship itself.[2]

In nationwide studies, according to patients and their physicians, this relationship consists, fundamentally, of three elements: compassion, understanding, and partnership.[5] While science, technology, and competence are recognized as essential and enabling, they are quite separate from the core elements of the relationship, which work in unison to support mutual confidence, trust, and respect.[5]

Understanding the relationship is critical if one is to correct what has been a defective value proposition in health care. For almost two decades, value has been defined as quality over cost. Quality refers to measurable and quantifiable, outcomes-measured, protocol-driven, evidence-based quality. Cost is tied to processes and resources. The logic has been that as processes are re-engineered and simplified, costs will decline, outcomes will be more reliable, and safety advanced.[2]

In advancing measurable quality, most agree that progress has been made, at least for those insured Americans. It is clear, as well, that until recently, cost has been better managed. And yet, through this active period of health care redesign, heavily centered on a concept of managed care delivered by HMOs, majorities of physicians and patients have withheld support because they did not see the output as valuable.[6]

To understand why, we need only return to the definition of our health system's core relationship. The patient-physician relationship is compassion, understanding, and partnership, in both clinical care and educational empowerment. This output fundamentally requires a key ingredient: participation, which in turn requires time and a personalized encounter. This was left unaccounted for in the original value equation. Had policy experts been basing value redesign decisions on the correct equation—that is, value in health care equals quality over cost plus participation—it is likely we would be further along in our health system evolution, with stronger support from both patients and physicians.[4]

A second core issue, left unaddressed and ignored, is the issue of equity. Gro Brundtland, former head of the World Health Organization, defined care as goodness—that is, the highest quality, outcome-driven care—and fairness, or care delivered equitably across a population. In a first-of-its-kind comparison of worldwide health care systems based on five criteria, the United States ranked a sad 37th, not because of goodness or quality and expertise, but because of fairness or equitable distribution of care and resources to our population. An employer-based health insurance system, with urban and rural pockets of poverty, and an inadequate safety net reliant on the goodwill of physicians, nurses, and hospitals, has become frayed and broken. This not only creates a crisis of conscience, but also ensures that our goal of moving from intervention to prevention, from hospital-based to home-based, from paternalism to partnership, from individual approaches to team-based approaches, from disability to productivity, and from disintegration to integration will be a rocky road indeed.

The solution must be anchored in the fundamental philosophy of goodness and fairness in health care. Upon this base we are able to support the weight of scientific integrity, adequate resources, and a commitment to equity. Properly grounded, areas of concentration naturally evolve, including education and training, cross-sector cooperation, and wise leveraging of technology. A commitment to evidence-based medicine, to grassroots decision-making, and access—to caregivers and the wide range of diagnostic and therapeutic discoveries—becomes a natural progression, delivering quality, cost control, and participation. In this environment, the relationship-based care system can flourish, and at the end of the day citizens and their caregivers will declare the systems and their services valuable.

7.
Managing Chronic Disease in the Home

As populations age in the United States, the absence of lifecycle health planning to prevent disease and ineffectual management of chronic illnesses which already exist create an uncertain medical future. First, let's consider our current burden of disease. By 2030, a fifth of the U.S. population will be over 65, and many will face the challenges of managing one or more chronic illnesses for a significant number of years, including physical and psychological distress, functional dependency and frailty, and a need for support.[1]

Traditional care systems are not particularly well-equipped for this situation. For example, our medical system focuses almost exclusively on curing illnesses and prolonging life—goals shaped by the hard-charging interventional past. But in the new order, these two worthwhile goals become hollow if they're not pursued simultaneously with goals of improving quality of life, relieving suffering, and providing physical and emotional comfort.[2]

The palliative care movement addresses this concern. Palliative care, which focuses on supporting the needs of the chronically ill as they approach the final phase of life, is as much a home-based life philosophy and value position as it is a caring revolution. Two leaders of the movement recently noted: "The aim of palliative care is to relieve suffering and improve the quality of life for patients with advanced illnesses and support their families."[1]

The process of getting there is as important as the goal itself. Palliative care calls for an extraordinarily inclusive team effort with a strong emphasis on planning.

This philosophy of care begins with physicians eliciting the concerns of the patient and loved ones. What is important in the patient's life? What more would he or she like to achieve? Is there something he or she fears worse than death?[3]

Concerns expressed during this conversation help define the patient's value system. Studies have found that patients almost always express the desire for more effective communication with a care team that is comfortable dealing with uncertainty and complexity. It's important for the care team to tailor care to the patient's individual needs.[4]

Palliative care is remarkably focused and pragmatic. If I place myself in an elder patient's shoes—multiple diseases, some compromise in capacity, and an uncertain prognosis—priorities become more obvious. What would I need? What would I ask of my caregivers? First, relieve my suffering. Second, improve the quality of my life. Third, manage my pain and other symptoms effectively over a long span. Fourth, while you are caring for me physically, don't abandon me psychologically or spiritually. Help me grieve my losses. Fifth, be sure to coordinate this as a team effort, remembering that my family and I are part of the team.

At the end of the day, the patient seeks enough comfort to contribute to loved ones' lives, enough resources to not be a burden to family and friends, and enough strength and capacity to control one's own life.[5]

Many people are dealing with these issues with their loved ones now, but it makes good sense to plan ahead for a time when this generation will have multiple medical conditions themselves but will not yet be in the dying process.

Where do hospice services fit in with palliative care? Hospice care has a remarkable track record in supportive, holistic, end-of-life care. In the United States, however, it has been primarily associated with terminal care of cancer patients and those with end-stage chronic diseases like Alzheimer's. Insurance coverage for hospice services requires physician certification that a patient has only six months to live. Such certification in non-cancer chronic diseases is increasingly common.[6]

Slowly, around the world, care systems are beginning to absorb the teachings of hospice in the form of chronic-disease management, team coordination, and a holistic, patient -and home-centered care approach. When successful outcomes are well-defined, everyone benefits. For example, patients should be able to voice their personal needs and define their long-term and short-term goals. Evaluation should be thorough on the front end and take into account what patients define as an excellent outcome. Care should be well-planned, based on these expectations, and discussions should be summarized in treatment plans and treatment directives, leaving little to chance. And a trusted health care proxy should be identified, in case the patient becomes incapable of making his or her own health decisions. With this road map, care execution and coordination manage the complexity of the situation, helping to simplify a patient's remaining time.[1]

When palliative care plans are successful, what do we find? More joy and pleasure; less pain and worry. We also find less hospitalization, fewer nursing home placements, greater patient and family satisfaction, greater caregiver health and well-being, and, in the end, a greater likelihood of a peaceful death, surrounded by loved ones, at home.[1]

None are more challenged by health complexity than those confronting Alzheimer's disease or adult dementia. The incidence of Alzheimer's disease in the United States is on a steep rise. Over the next 50 years we'll see a 300 percent increase in affected patients. In 2000, there were 4.5 million Americans with the disease. This number will increase to nearly 6 million by 2020, nearly 8 million by 2030, and top 13 million in 2050.[7]

With the increase in patients comes a predictable increase in costs. Some of those costs are very visible and trackable. For example, it is projected that direct costs to Medicare for Alzheimer's will increase 54 percent to $49 billion in 2010. Medicaid, which carries the burden of nursing home payments, is expected to expend $33 billion, an 80 percent increase, by 2010 for Alzheimer's patients.[7]

But this only begins to tell the financial story, because the larger burden is hidden in the indirect impact of Alzheimer's.[8, 9] For example, it is projected that the annual cost to business this year in indirect outlays related to Alzheimer's patients will top $60 billion,with $37 billion tied to lost caregiver productivity.[7] This reflects the reality that the majority of care is provided by family members. In a recent study, the average age of caregivers was 65, while the average age of patients was 81. More than 80 percent of the caregivers were women family members. Of that number, half were children of patients and the other half were spouses of patients.[10]

Caring for patients with significant cognitive impairment is challenging at best. Let's begin with the extraordinary length of the disease—an average of eight years, which can feel like an eternity. During those years, loved ones disappear before your eyes, but they don't go quietly. The level of impairment is extreme, requiring early support with the basics. More than half of caregivers spend an average 11 hours a week on basic activities of daily living (ADLs) and an additional 35 hours a week on instrumental activities of daily living (IADLs).[10]

The time required to provide care amounts to a full-time job. Over 50 percent in one study averaged 46 hours a week of care. And a similar number felt they were "on-call" 24 hours a day without relief. The impact is rapid and direct, with the clearest evidence being caregivers' abandonment of their regular jobs. Forty-eight percent decrease their regular work hours, and 18 percent resign from their regular jobs.[10]

But that's only what you see. Here's what you don't see. The rates of depression in caregivers are significant. Fully 43 percent of caregivers of Alzheimer's patients in one study were clinically depressed.[10] And only the death of the patient brings lasting relief. Seventeen percent of these caregivers require anti-depressant medicine and 19 percent require anti-anxiety medications. These rates do not decline if the patient is placed in a nursing home, leaving the family caregiver to struggle with the guilt of abandonment, concerns over institutional care, and bereavement for a loved one who is lost but not gone. It is only after a patient dies, with an average of three to 12 months of recovery, that depression levels in family caregivers decline to below the levels of depression that existed when they were active caregivers.[10, 11]

So the reality is pretty clear-cut. While unpaid family caregivers of Alzheimer's patients spare the government direct expenses of institutionalization, this does not come without a cost. Equally clear is that patients prefer to be at home, and caregivers receive no mental relief by providing home care. Finally, we know that this complex crisis for the American family will get worse rapidly in our immediate future.

What can be done? The solution lies in better systems for home-based support for patients and caregivers. This has the potential to increase quality of care and decrease cost of care. Experts suggest these services focus on five key areas: Advanced communication connectivity to address social isolation; pain control; technology enabled vigilance or oversight of wandering behavior; counseling and positive reinforcement for caregivers; and health team-based inclusion long-term support of caregivers.[12]

If America's health insurers—government and private—are looking for worthwhile home-based projects on which to collaborate, incentivizing our movement toward palliative care approaches for chronic disease management, and support for the caregivers of Alzheimer's and dementia patients might be an excellent place to start.

8.
Long Distance Caregiving

For families of seniors with Alzheimer's disease and other chronic diseases, colliding megatrends are increasingly pitting family loyalties against workplace loyalties. If you think it is hard to care for a chronically ill family member at home, try it from a distance. As the U.S. population has aged, families have become more mobile, separated by geography, and occupied by work demands. Large numbers of women have entered the workplace, and global competitiveness has placed increasing emphasis on worker retention and productivity. Thus, family caregiving from a distance has become a fact of life for millions of Americans, according to a recent survey commissioned by MetLife Mature Market Institute and the National Alliance for Caregiving.[1]

Approximately 34 million Americans are providing care to older family members. Fifteen percent of these caregivers live an hour or more away from their relative. Nearly one-fourth of these long-distance caregivers are the only or the primary care provider, and 80 percent work part- or full-time, according to the MetLife survey of 1,130 long-distance family care providers.[1,2]

Long-distance caregivers provide a wide array of services at great cost to themselves. According to the survey, they spend an average of $392 per month—about half of this is spent on out-of-pocket purchases and services for the care recipient and half on travel and long-distance communications.[1]

The expenditure in time is no less than the expenditure in dollars. Half of the survey respondents reported spending 13.6 hours a month arranging care services, and half said they spend another 16 hours a month checking on their care recipient or monitoring the care being received. Nearly three-quarters of these long-distance caregivers provide help with Instrumental Activities of Daily Living (IADLs) such as transportation, shopping, cooking, cleaning, managing finances and medications—for an average of 22 hours per month. And 40 percent are involved in basic Activities of Daily Living (ADLs) such as bathing, dressing, feeding, and toileting, for an average of 12 hours per month.[1]

What effect does long-distance caregiving have on professional work schedules? Employed caregivers are often required to make significant adjustments to allow for their caregiving responsibilities. These include coming in late or leaving early, missing days of work, rearranging work schedules, and taking unpaid leave. Twenty-five percent of the surveyed long-distance caregivers had shortened their workday and 36 percent reported missing full days of work. Twelve percent had taken a leave of absence.[1]

Distance, of course, makes a difference in the work accommodations caregivers make. Those caregivers who live closer to the care recipient are more likely to come into work late or leave early, as opposed to missing full workdays.[1]

The forces that have created today's long-distance caregiver realities are unlikely to reverse themselves in the near future. Rather, the challenges and work-balance issues are likely to accelerate. Clearly, long-distance caregiving already impacts retention and productivity. Physical distance is a key determinant in terms of complexity, as is the presence or absence of other relatives in the area. In the absence of "on-the-ground" family support, paid support becomes more critical earlier in the aging cycle.[1,2]

What can an employer do? Certainly, sensitizing line managers to the issue is a reasonable starting point. Adjusting policies to allow job sharing and short-time relief, as well as providing information and help in coordinating eldercare, are definitely worthwhile investments, compared with the cost of attrition and lost productivity. And, since long-distance caregivers have financial burdens as well as time conflicts, programs that offer help with these are beneficial. For example, voluntary pooling of frequent flyer miles for employees who need to travel on family emergencies is an idea worth considering.[1,3]

These tangible expressions of support face the issue head-on while reinforcing shared values and joint commitment. Still the risks of caring from a distance are real. Take for example the issue of elder abuse. As Stephanie Lederman, executive director of the American Federation for Aging Research, notes, "A large segment of our population is both dependent and frail. Studies on elder abuse now alert us that seniors are also vulnerable and in need of help."[4]

And the problem is getting worse. According to the most recent study from the National Center on Elder Abuse, the incidence rate of elder abuse increased 150 percent between 1986 and 1996.[5]

How large is the at-risk segment? One study of 2,812 adults over age 65 revealed that 6 percent, or 176, of them were seen by elderly protective services over a nine-year period. Nearly three-quarters of these cases involved self-neglect, but the remaining 27 percent were traced to the actions of others —nearly 6 percent of the elderly people experienced physical abuse, 17 percent had been neglected, and almost 5 percent suffered exploitation.[6]

What is elder abuse? The U.S. National Academy of Sciences defines the problem as "intentional actions that cause harm or create a serious risk of harm to a vulnerable elder by a caregiver or other person who stands in a trust relationship to the elder; or, failure by a caregiver to satisfy the elder's basic needs or to protect the elder from harm."[7]

Elder abuse not only implies that a person has suffered injury or neglect, but also that a specific individual, entrusted to provide care, is responsible. The abuse may take a variety of forms, including physical abuse, psychological abuse, sexual assault, exploitation of material resources, or neglect.

Studying elder abuse is easier said than done. For example, a simple geriatric study on how to prevent elder fractures due to falls must consider confounding issues such as polypharmacy, visual impairment from cataracts and other conditions, and depression or dementia, to name a few.[8] When one then attempts to decipher naturally occurring injuries from deliberate ones, study design and verification become critical. Was an injury due to loss of balance or assault? Did weight loss occur due to chronic disease and cancer or from neglect? Was under- or overmedicating the result of forgetfulness or malevolence of the caregiver?[8,9]

Risk factors associated with elder abuse are increasingly clear. Most incidences occur in shared living situations where there is prolonged access by a family member, friend, or entrusted surrogate. Elder dementia creates both a complex management challenge and an unreliable witness to the abuse, which complicates documentation. Social isolation creates stress that can lead to reactive abuse behavior, as well as a hidden environment to harbor abuse, neglect, or exploitation. The presence of caregiver mental illness, including depression or substance abuse, increases the likelihood of harmful behaviors, as does the use of family-member caregivers who are dependent upon and often resentful of the senior for whom they are charged to provide care.[6,9]

Caring for a frail, dependent, and vulnerable senior is challenging under the best circumstances. When abuse is interjected, the consequences are significant, including an increase in mortality rates. One study has documented that the three-year mortality rate for seniors who are exposed to elder abuse was 91 percent, compared with 58 percent in a matched dependent senior population that was not abused.[6]

Dr. Mark Lachs and his colleagues note, "It seems plausible that experiencing elder abuse is an extreme form of negative social support. In the same manner that social integration reduces mortality, it may conversely be the case that the extreme interpersonal stress resulting from elder abuse situations may confer additional death risk."[6]

Screening elders for abuse requires high awareness and good clinical judgment. There is not a clear consensus on routine monitoring or an instrument to be used.[6,9] General concern should be raised when physicians, nurses, and other members of the care team observe a poor social network, poor social functioning, and signs of conflict between a patient and a caregiver. Clinicians should trust their clinical judgment and instincts, do a complete physical assessment with a focus on cognitive function, question the patient in private, and be cautious in discussions with the caregiver, extending empathy while uncovering the individual's mental status and coping skills.[9]

Similarly, families should trust their instincts. Is mom or dad declining without an obvious reason? What is the level of cleanliness of the patient and the home setting? What is the patient being fed, and, under direct viewing, how gentle and effective is the process? Are there unexplained bruises, blisters, or painful areas? Is the senior's mobility rapidly declining? What is being said to the senior, not simply with words, but also with messages and tone? And what do your instincts tell you when you make unannounced visits?

Addressing senior abuse requires a continuum of committed individuals from home to care sites and back home again, providing reliable monitoring, oversight, diagnosis, and intervention when necessary. Such a network must be built, and a good place to begin is with an informed discussion of the issue between family members and their care teams.

9.
New Entrants in Health Care

The challenge of managing, often from a distance, an aging population burdened with chronic diseases is real enough. But our parallel challenge, and the only way to end this destructive cycle of chronic disease and disability, is to leverage technology to build out a system of health planning and health performance that begins at birth and extends out 100 years or more—a truly preventive health care effort.

For many caregivers of my generation, technology has been viewed with double suspicion. First has been our concern that it would separate us from the people we serve, undermining touch and trust. Second has been the worry that technology in the wrong hands could drive policy in the wrong direction—limiting choice, access, coverage, privacy, and relationships between the people and the people caring for the people.

But now a year short of 60, I see, even in my own peers, and certainly in the two younger generations of new clinicians rising in the ranks, a greater sense of security about technology, a belief that it can be harnessed for good; but to do so, physicians, nurses, and other caregivers must be in front of this movement and define it.

This requires not simply an understanding of the interface between science and technology, but also a broad and impassioned view of what we would like to build out as a better health care system and an understanding of how best to utilize technology as a connector, informer, and enabler to get us there effectively and efficiently.

Some of the steps that are pointing us toward a better way to approach health have become increasingly obvious. These include:

- Re-centering the health care system around multigenerational prevention and healthy homes.

- Moving from electronic medical records (EMRs) to personal health records (PHRs) and from personal health records to lifespan planning records (LPRs)

- Empowering and connecting health consumers and supporting their active engagement and full participation in health care teams.

- Expanding coverage to all and critically examining the wisdom of an employer-based, nontransportable health insurance system.

- Moving diagnosis of chronic disease from age 60 to age 20, and adherence to treatment plans from under 50% to over 75%.

In all of the above, technologic advances in information, engineering and science are in the process of being harnessed, and if done well, could assist the United States. In applying its vast national spending in health care in a more effective, equitable, and just manner. But, to do so, caring professionals of my generation must allow themselves to become excited about the possibilities of leveraging technology and involved in reshaping the system itself.

What if, for example, you were able to place sensors in the orthotic shoes of diabetics, and if they and their clinicians could be alerted when pressure levels reached a point where the possibility of developing a skin breakdown was imminent. How many of the 90,000 diabetic amputations in the U.S. populations 21 million diabetics could be prevented? Imagine the savings in suffering and dollars, and the increases in productivity. Well, companies are working on that, patents have been filed, and new products will launch this year and next.[1]

And what if we had a simple multi-gene test that could identify the 20 percent of lung cancer patients who truly would benefit from chemotherapy? That would revolutionize our staging system for this disease. Well, reported in the *New England Journal of Medicine*, National Taiwan University's Hsuan-Ya Chen and his colleagues have devised such a test.[2]

And what if GE, or Siemens, or Intel, or Microsoft really went after re-engineering the home, so that it wasn't simply "where the heart is" but also becomes "where the health is;" and what if they simultaneously recognized that the Lifespan Planning Record (LPR) is the killer application that will finally tip America's health care system from intervention to prevention? That would be exciting, right?

To succeed in building out such a vision, traditional health care leaders must reach out and partner with innovators who have not traditionally been associated with the leading edge of health delivery. Who are the non-traditional players entering the health care space? The four most active on the horizon are technology firms, entertainment firms, financial firms, and governmental municipalities.

The technology firms have been fast at work, somewhat below the radar screen, developing a wide range of products to re-outfit the home for health and expand connectivity. Some of them—big names like Intel and Philips—have linked hands with leaders in the aging-services community to form CAST (the Center for Aging Services Technologies) and have recently broadened their vision to embrace physicians, nurses, informal family caregivers, and multigenerational lifespan health planning.[3,4]

Not to be left out, entertainment firms have entered the health space with enthusiasm. Where? Well, pretty much everywhere. Google is in health decision-making through its search engines. YouTube carries health videos, including my own Health Politics which had nearly 300,000 video downloads in 2006. MySpace sees the potential to be the self-help, health platform, and isolation buster of the future. And it goes on and on.

The financial industry has entered health on the back of Health Savings Accounts, known as HSAs. Hundreds of financial services companies have been drawn in by the promise of lucrative fees they can generate with maintenance and transaction charges, and more significantly, by offering consumers various investment vehicles as their HSA balances grow. In fact, collectively, HSA balances could reach $75 billion in the coming years.[5]

So it's no wonder as banks have entered health that many insurers are creating or becoming banks. UnitedHealthcare was the first to create a bank in 2002, and BlueCross BlueShield followed suit two years later.[6, 7] As insurers develop their new role in the transitioning system, it remains to be seen whether or not they will fundamentally reinforce or put up barriers to the whole idea.

I'm talking about their historic love/hate relationship with the patient-physician relationship—a key part of a preventive health care system. Insurers currently play a major role, sometimes reinforcing connectivity, other times positioning the people in opposition to their caregivers—and physicians and hospitals in opposition to each other—in attempts to hold down costs. It is also unclear at this point whether the financial services firms will primarily align with care providers as they expand into health, as the technology groups have, or primarily align with insurers.

What does appear clear, however, is that the primitive state of our health information infrastructure, which has frustrated traditional health care leaders for some time now, is viewed by both financial and technology firms as an opportunity rather than an obstacle. Out of our current situation, they envision delivering success in the short term by leveraging their unique skills and experience in information systems and data management, utilizing their existent information architecture, and investing some of their vast financial resources.

The federal government has also weighed in. In 2001, an advisory committee to the Department of Health and Human Services put together a vision and planning report for a National Health Information Infrastructure (NHII).[8] In 2003, the Department of Health and Human Services organized a national consensus meeting to gather the opinions of 580 expert participants. All the key health care system stakeholders were represented. And, in 2004, the results from this conference were reported.[9]

Where did they find agreement? First, in the deliverables. A national health information superhighway is required to improve patient care, triggering and enabling not only modern information management, but also process re-engineering to reduce errors and variability and increase safety. Beyond acute care, the information highway would improve management of chronic diseases by promoting consistently high standards of care and allowing home monitoring with facilitated patient-clinician communications. Patient education would be expanded and individualized, and would support behavioral change. Databases, secured for privacy, would allow population research as well as public health surveillance for conditions like SARS.[9]

National leadership, cross-sector resourcing, and community-based participation is slowly coalescing to tackle these manageable challenges. The consensus committee has recommended 40 to 50 demonstration projects, many now underway, centered on key principles, including maintenance of confidentiality, non-proprietary status, national scalability, easy-to-use technology, low barriers to entry, standardization that ensures compatibility and connectivity, and support of the patient-physician relationship.[9]

As for municipal governments, they're not waiting around either, though their entry into health is largely subconscious and part of a broader set of competitive objectives. Witness San Francisco as a case-in-point, with its 760,000 residents and additional 400,000 weekly commuters. Following the lead of Philadelphia and proceeding in tandem with other large cities like Chicago and Boston, San Francisco has completed the first step in creating a citywide wireless network with free access that blankets the city's 49 square miles.

In April 2006, the city announced the selection of Google and Earthlink, working with Tropos Networks and Motorola, to build out the wireless network. A primary goal is to equitably address and eliminate any digital divide by providing wireless access to residents who might not otherwise be able to get it.[9]

When completed, all citizens will have the opportunity to utilize free service from Google at a rate that is six times faster than a dial-up connection, with some on-screen advertising. Earthlink service will also be provided, without advertising, at four times the connection speed of the Google offering, for $20 per month. It's anticipated that most citizens will use Google, while most small business will use Earthlink. A vigorous public debate around commercialization and pricing is currently focused on whether to allow the companies to track "cookies," the identifiers that define type of usage and enable customized electronic delivery of ads—an issue of privacy.[10]

Ten million dollars will be spent in the San Francisco build out, and 70 times that is expected to be spent on similar projects nationwide over the next three years.[10] And it's not just big cities. Hundreds of at-risk small communities, from rural Native American tribes to impoverished Appalachian communities aided by university development grants are busy creating their own WiMax (think WiFi on steroids) networks that can now extend WiFi low-cost wireless access across a 50-mile radius.[11] At the same time, many other projects, such as the one targeting Atlanta Hawks season ticket holders in 2006 (conducted by Nokia, Cingular, Chase, and Visa) are converging technologies to allow electronic transactions with hand-held devices. For these fans, that means being able to order and pay for concessions using their cell phones, which are linked to their Visa credit cards, and receiving "just-in-time" proprietary sports information designed exclusively for them.[12]

With this kind of technology in place, it doesn't take much to envision cities with robust and reliable wireless health care communications networks in place – allowing transmission of critical data back and forth between patients and health care providers to assist shared decision-making.

So let's put it all together. One, the new health care system will be centered in the home, with the primary information loop going from home to care team and back to home. It will manage chronic disease and preventive lifespan planning simultaneously, attempting to capture the learnings from the former to inform and improve the latter. Two, build-out requires a pervasive, standardized information highway and new devices to generate the necessary diagnostic and medical information and easily transmit it to trusted caregivers and advisers. Some of this build-out may not have been originally intended to support health care, but has the capacity to support a preventive system's daily needs. Three, traditional health sector players have demonstrated an inability to fund and build out such a system, focusing on the hospital-office interface and de-emphasizing the home. Four, technology, entertainment, and financial institutions are entering health in ways traditional health players either cannot or will not, and share three things in common: vast financial assets, enormous information technology expertise, and an existing presence in the home. Five, the federal government and local governmental municipalities are laying the technological groundwork and standards that will connect all the sectors and broaden the reach and impact of a new "wired" health care system.

If these new players can rapidly build out a health information loop that has broad, equitable reach and reinforces the connection between the people and their physician-led care teams, they will be richly rewarded. And we could all be healthier and happier in the new environment.

10.
Lifespan Planning Records

I f we allow ourselves to dream of a better health care system—one that permits us to feel connected, supported, and in control of our own health destiny—two words come to mind: information and planning. The more information we have about our own health history and genetic profile, the smarter we can be about making health decisions and planning our health future. This requires a constantly available "record" of our changing health status. But if you switch physicians or go to a hospital for surgery, you'll find that our nation's health records are not even close to this ideal. They are splintered and poorly organized at best. To their credit, physicians and hospitals have been trying to create a coordinated system of electronic records—but it falls far short of what we need.

The real key to our health information future is a concept called a "Lifespan Planning Record." This computer-based and integrated model would provide a holistic view of your health—stretching all the way back to your ancestors and projecting far forward into your future—so you will know what you can anticipate as your body ages. It helps define health as much more than the absence of illness. It's about life fulfillment.

With lifespan planning, we can start to concentrate on preventive activities in health—which is just about all that the experts say must happen if we are to fix our broken health care system. It will also make our health care system safer because the information we use will be more reliable. Don Detmer, President of the American Medical Informatics Association, said it best: "Significant improvements in health care safety and quality will not be achieved for Americans without robust, secure electronic health records within a national health information infrastructure."[1]

Implementing lifespan planning records won't be easy. As you can imagine, there are large technological and logistical hurdles. But we can at least start to sort out what some of the issues are. Let's have a look. The first thing you should know is that some of health care's most important players are spending significant time on the question of record-keeping—from the American Medical Informatics Association to The Robert Wood Johnson Foundation to the Agency for Healthcare Research and Quality.[2] Much of the challenge for groups like these is in determining how to build a system around what is, essentially, a moving target. Which parts of the plan should be derived from technology of the present, technology of the future, and technology from the distant future?

To adequately address those questions, let's look at the trends. First, longer life spans are moving us from three-generation families to four- and five-generation families—with more complicated health management needs.[3] Second, the health consumer movement is in full swing, with consumers carving out a more empowered role and demanding reform.[4] And third, information technology is advancing to provide new linkages between patient and caregiver and mind-boggling possibilities for data storage and exchange.[5] As these trends intersect, they are rapidly changing the very drawing board that is being used to plan for a new national health record system.

Here's what I mean: Over the last decade, the discussion about health care records has focused on electronic medical records—or EMRs—and aspired to improve accuracy and efficiency by converting paper-based systems used by physicians, nurses, and hospitals to electronic formats.[6] That's a worthy goal. But as leaders diligently began this conversion, the environment began to shift under foot—thanks largely to our three intersecting trends. In fact, by 2005 it had become quite clear to many leaders in the field that "The Record" properly resided with the patient from whom health data emerged, and that the data that flowed through the hands of hospitals, doctors and nurses was only a part of the overall picture. Thus the concept of a "personal health record" is gradually subsuming the vision of an electronic medical record.[7] This is a good development. The personal health record combines data, knowledge, and software tools, which help patients become participants in their health care. But if we are truly to anticipate where health care trends are taking us, even this is not enough.

It is now clear that in a truly preventive system, "health" is not a collection of late-stage, reactive interventions. That kind of thinking will soon be a relic of the past.[8] Rather, health should be defined as a life fully lived—hopeful, productive, fulfilling, rewarding, and manageable. The determinants of such a life begin before birth, embedded in the healthful behaviors of one's future parents, and they extend beyond death to ones' survivors. Considering this broader view of health, the right concept for our health record system should be a Lifespan Planning Record—or LPR. The LPR for a single individual born today could extend out at least 100 years. It would include all of the baseline medical information needed by patients, and much more. It would consider economic, social, educational, and spiritual goals and milestones as well as medical and scientific objectives.

Born today, the newborn child's plan would already be inhabited with a great deal of data. Some reasonable compilation of the records of parents, grandparents, and siblings would be represented. Future diagnostic and preventive therapeutic measures, based on familial information, would be flagged on the timeline. Print, video, and graphic information from other accessible intelligence databases would be seamlessly interwoven for easy use by the people caring for each other and this new global citizen. As time passes, this "living record" would flexibly grow and adjust to assist informed decision-making, preventive behavior, and full and complete human development.[9]

Where will the knowledge come from? Patients, obviously, will need to contribute to the personal side of the record. On the health and science side, it will emerge from three electronic data sources: the Clinical Research data space, the Continuing Professional Development data space, and the Continuing Consumer Education data space. These data sources will desegregate and converge to allow integrated use of the information they contain, by the people, the people caring for the people, and investigators searching for new solutions to today's unresolved problems.[10]

Obviously, many issues will need to be sorted out—not the least of which are confidentiality, patient privacy, and control over records. But the bottom line is that as quickly as the electronic medical record is being subsumed by the personal health record, the personal health record is now being subsumed by the need for a lifespan planning record— because that's the best way to move us toward a preventive care system.

11.

Making a Health Plan and Sticking to It

S tudies show that physicians have largely embraced partnerships with their patients. The days of "doctor says" and "patient does" are steadily drifting into the past. In concert, one-on-one strategies are giving way to team approaches as physicians begin to acknowledge that managing both clinical and educational continuums in support of educationally empowered health consumers requires a supportive team and delegation. "Doctor's orders" are increasingly being supplemented by mutual decision-making. The long-term goal: prevention rather than intervention.[1,2]

But we're not there yet. Why not? Part of the answer is our inability to reliably execute treatment plans. One indicator of this structural disconnect is the tension that has arisen over the language we use to describe patient execution and follow-through. Prior to the emergence of health consumerism, the Internet, and prevention-focused medicine, health care leaders spoke often of compliance: the extent to which a patient follows medical instructions. Today we look at adherence: the extent to which a person's behavior—taking medication, following a diet, or executing lifestyle changes—corresponds with agreed recommendations from a health caregiver.[3,4]

Changes in language often signal the onset of process and system redesign. Recent publications by the World

Health Organization and the American Medical Association have made it clear that adherence is a worldwide issue that will grow in significance with aging of our populations and coincident increases in the prevalence of chronic diseases.[4,5] The WHO report notes, "In developed countries, adherence among patients suffering chronic diseases averages only 50 percent." And the challenge is greater in the developing world. For example, studies show that adherence to treatment regimens for hypertension are 51 percent in the United States, 43 percent in China, but only 27 percent in Gambia.[4] Studies also reveal that the developing world is rapidly encountering a dual burden of disease as it confronts infectious diseases and malnutrition on the one hand, and marketing-driven behavioral changes that increase tobacco use, poor nutrition, and subsequently the incidence of chronic diseases and cancer on the other.[6]

The reasons for poor adherence are well-understood, but the solutions are only now taking shape. Adherence requires that a patient fully understand and comprehend the plan, be in full agreement with the course of action, and be committed to the execution of what is increasingly a multistep solution.[7] Thinking for a moment just about medication therapy for a well-motivated, engaged patient with resources, what questions would be required to generate baseline information? Here are just a few: How much medication is needed? How often? Same time every day? Do I empty the bottle? Do I need a refill? Side effects? Will I become addicted? Any interactions with my other medicines? Do you have information I can take with me? Whom do I call if I have a problem? And that doesn't even begin to address more substantive lifestyle behavioral changes.

The reality is that ensuring adherence is complex. No single strategy has been known to be effective.[4] What we do know is that good follow-through is a local phenomenon and is most likely if interventions are tailored to the individual patients; if patients are supported rather than blamed; and if patients, families, and communities are actively involved.

Peer support can be critical according to the WHO report, which says, "There is substantial evidence that peer support among patients can improve adherence to therapy while reducing the amount of time devoted by the health professionals to the care of chronic conditions."[4]

Measuring adherence remains problematic. The WHO report continues, "There is no 'gold standard' for measuring adherence behavior ... measurement of adherence remains only an estimate of a patient's actual behavior."[4] But technology, in the form of future "smart" delivery systems that use the detection of chemical signals in the body to release appropriate dosages from internalized reservoirs of medicine are on the horizon.[7] Cross-sector partnerships are also beginning to attack behavioral change and chronic diseases in a more deliberate and multi-year manner with some success.[8]

Is the investment worth it? Economists would say "without a doubt." In the United States alone, the annual cost of poor adherence is estimated at $75 billion to $100 billion. The human cost is even more striking—125,000 preventable deaths and 10 percent to 25 percent of all hospital and nursing home admissions.[7] As Dr. Eduardo Sabaté, medical officer of the WHO, has noted, "Better adherence will not threaten health care budgets. On the contrary, adherence will result in a significant decrease in the overall health budget. This is due to the reduction in the need for more costly interventions, unnecessary use of emergency room services, and highly expensive intensive care services."[4]

In addition to financial benefits, the medical benefits are real, including fewer medical complications, better quality of life, decreases in antibiotic drug resistance, wiser use of limited health resources, decreases in pain and intervention, and increases in workforce productivity.[4,7] Former U.N. Secretary-General Kofi Annan perhaps said it best: "When we are sick, working is hard and learning is harder still. Illness blunts our creativity, cuts out opportunities."[4]

12.

Bringing Health Education into the Home

I n a recent panel discussion at a national medical meeting on the subject of health education, a panelist took the opportunity to bemoan the continued failure of broadcast television to accurately communicate and educate on a host of medical topics.[1] Yet, what the expert and the vast majority of the medical audience missed was that medical communications have now gone virtual; that in an age of prevention, health information support becomes the lead "health product"; and that what they discussed as the network's responsibility is actually a network of patients and families who are the physicians' responsibility.

Just over two decades ago, educational empowerment of health consumers began in earnest. Over the following years, the public's understanding of the scientific lexicon, of organ function (physiology), and of disease-caused dysfunction (pathophysiology) has gradually expanded. As an outflow of this growing health literacy, individuals, families, and communities are increasingly focused on wellness strategies, behavioral modification, treatment-plan adherence, and lifecycle management. The net goal: decrease intervention by increasing prevention. The expectation? That this front-end investment of time and effort might increase quality of life, productivity, earning power, cost-effectiveness, and societal well-being.[2]

Yet most national and state medical organizations are very early in the process of fleshing out an implementable set of low- and high-tech strategies that would accomplish real-time, bidirectional information support with their "local network of patients"—a network that begins with the patient in the home, extends to the physician and other care team members, and then loops back to home; a network that integrates nurses, hospitals, and health care systems; a network that closely coordinates continuing medical education with continuing consumer education and attacks translational gaps; and, finally, an advanced communication network, not led by NBC, CBS, ABC, or CNN, but by the physicians, nurses, and care teams.

Such a network considers information generation, distribution, analysis, and feedback. Process design, practice monitors, and measured outcomes drive network improvement. In addition, a physician-led patient informational network must address complex policy issues including privacy, confidentiality, network security, liability, financing, and reimbursement.

In simplest terms, the patient-education network aims to connect home to care team at a time when both are actively evolving. By 2015, many homes will have pervasive networked computers feeding into intelligence software, measuring behaviors against predictive health behavior models.[3] Physician-supported coaching interfaces will cue, remind, and encourage by phone, TV, radio, or iPod-like gadgets that will be a third of the size and a 10th of the cost they are now.[4] Data from patient-monitored activities and a myriad of new diagnostic instruments will stream vital signs, blood results, and imaging from the home to the care team, who will analyze, document, and communicate back to the patient and be reimbursed for the same.[5]

Within this advanced medical communications network, patient inclusion will be the rule. Not only will patients continuously dialogue with their physicians and caregivers, but they will also dialogue—endorsed and encouraged by their care team—with each other, creating customized in-network self-help teams that aggressively attack social isolation. The communication network will be highly personalized, fully advantaging the varied skill sets, values, and reach of nurses and other health professionals. It will preserve financial capital while expanding human, social, and cultural capital.

Is this notion of a micro-medical network unrealistic or too far off to make it practical for serious strategy planning now? The simple answer is no. But as Dr. Claude Lenfant, former director of the National Institutes of Health writes, "Moving the knowledge off the shelves and into practice, making it relevant and accessible to practitioners and patients, achieving a true marriage of knowledge with intuition and judgment—all this requires translation."[6]

But the reality is that the eyes of patients and doctors alike are frequently on the future rather than the present. Seventy-two percent of Americans believe that new scientific and medical breakthroughs are essential for staying healthy.[7] Yet the Institute of Medicine report in 2003 pulls us back to the present with this comment: "The stark reality is that we spend billions in research to find appropriate treatments...but we repeatedly fail to translate that knowledge and capacity into clinical practice."[8]

The truth is, we have trouble moving knowledge off the shelf and down the "translational highway."[9] This is not surprising when you look at the major stops along the way. Basic science must give way to clinical research studies. The studies must weave through the regulatory process to become approved therapies. The therapies must challenge the status quo to become the new standard of medical practice. And even if clinicians broadly adopt a new approach, patients must comply to yield positive outcomes.

There is no better example of the chasm between knowledge and practice than cardiovascular disease. "What we know" is frequently not "what we do." We know that beta-blockers used post-heart attack save lives. But a study in 1996—15 years after this discovery—showed only 62.5 percent of post-heart attack patients used this medication.[10] We know that all patients post-heart attack should be screened for cholesterol, but in reality only one-half to three-quarters of them are.[11] We know that aspirin is lifesaving for patients with coronary artery disease, and yet only one-third of them use aspirin.[12] And we know that patients with acute heart attack should receive clot-dissolving therapy or acute angioplasty, but only one-third of them do.[13]

Establishing and promoting professional standards of care can move the dial. The National Committee for Quality Assurance (NCQA), with its Health Plan Employer Data and Information Set (HEDIS), measures and informs practice in the majority of U.S. health plans. Significant improvement has occurred in NCQA members. For example, beta-blocker use post-heart attack has risen from 62.5 percent in 1996 to 92.5 percent in 2001. And appropriate use of blood pressure control medication has risen from 39 percent in 1999 to 55.4 percent in 2001.[14]

Patients seem poised to assume greater responsibility as well. A study in 2001 revealed that 94 percent of U.S. patients were more involved in health decisions, 92 percent took more control of their own health, and 82 percent had more discussions with physicians compared with ten years ago. Still, patients remain more focused on short-term than long-term benefits, with 93 percent willing to accept the risk of a prescription medicine if it will cure a disease, but only 49 percent willing to comply if it prevents a disease.[15]

Building a successful "translational highway" requires speaking to clinicians and patients simultaneously. Publications are an important first step, and fundamental to scientific exchange of ideas.[16] However, there are some 400,000 medical scientific articles per year, many more than even the most highly motivated clinician can absorb.[17] One strategy to manage this volume and complexity is the consensus conference: one or two days of highly focused discussion yielding consensus on a standard of care. Public education has also proven to be useful. For example, the

"Back to Sleep" campaign, encouraging parents to place infants to sleep on their backs to prevent Sudden Infant Death Syndrome (SIDS), resulted in a 43 percent decline in deaths from 1992 to 1997.[18] Consumer word of mouth, activated by voluntary health organizations, combines education and motivation. Advertising can help provide accurate information, consumer dialogue, and engagement between patients and physicians as we see in many "ask your doctor" campaigns. And finally, leveraging the patient-physician relationship to provide not only clinical support, but also educational support, can be highly effective.

We're slowly learning how to translate discovery into practice. But with an explosion of discoveries on the horizon and boomer aging just around the corner, we need to repave the "translational highway" and add a few lanes as well. Virtual health education—low cost, efficient, and direct—is uniquely positioned to broaden our health education highways. Increasingly built to standards, its components will be interchangeable and customizable, with caregivers drawing from content originating from varied sources.[19] Such flexibility and power in the hands of end-users will challenge traditional central-control models.

As health consumers become increasingly empowered and engaged, their many benefit/risk decision points will be jointly negotiated with their physicians.[20] This will be even more pronounced among informal caregivers who, as they achieve home health manager status, will be active members of the physician team.[21] These engaged consumers will expect access to the same knowledge support as other caregivers and will drive the development of Continuing Consumer Education (CCE) in parallel and often intersecting with Continuing Medical Education (CME). CCE will need to address their multiple expectations, including elimination of the translation gap, obliteration of "talking down," organized benefit/risk appraisal, expansion of their math literacy to manage basic statistics and prevalence data, and clear definition of the "knowns" and "unknowns" that caring professionals are often too reluctant to reveal.

Their demands for transparency in return for confidence and trust and their intolerance for translational delays will reshape public/private partnerships in CME. Think Google as well as Mayo Clinic. In fact, as demands for real-time, just-in-time CME and CCE gather speed, virtual CME will collapse down onto Clinical Research Databases, ultimately connecting the discovery industry on the one hand with patients and physicians in need of those discoveries on the other. [22]

Vertical CME, driven by medical elites, will give way to horizontal CME that is community-based. This will be disruptive to accrediting bodies, academic institutions and their experts, and the meeting industry and its sponsors. In the future, content will skip many of these steps, going direct to patients and their physicians, nurses, and caregivers in a manner that reinforces common visioning and strengthens the patient-physician relationship. Traditional peer review journals will adjust to these new realities, adapting existing vehicles and creating new, mostly electronic platforms that have the ability to translate and amplify less accessible existing medical informational products.

As CME becomes virtual, it will become one portion of a growing menu of offerings to support lifelong learning. Tomorrow's virtual education continuum is already popping up in bits and pieces today. It will include patient-specific decision-support research, virtual consultations, virtual CME, virtual class auditing, and virtual degrees (like MPHs) from full-fledged virtual universities like Hibernia College. It offers a masters in pharmaceutical medicine with Boston College, Harvard's Kennedy School, and the University of Dublin. [23]

In many ways, it is educational empowerment that has consummated the consumer revolution and sealed the new patient-physician relationship. As such, CME and CCE are now fully in the mix and well on their way to being "out of the box." Caring professionals, whether they know it or not, are on their way back into the home. And the horse that will ultimately carry them is health consumer education.

13.
Equity and Justice

For many Americans, there remains no health plan and no opportunity for adherence because there is no access. A health care safety net in the United States is not a luxury, but rather a necessity. It has become necessary because we chronically possess large numbers of uninsured as a result of our employer-based health insurance system. If you're out of work in America, it's a double hit. You lose your pay and your health insurance, and that's if you were lucky enough to be in a job that provided benefits.

What we call a safety net may not reliably catch you if you're uninsured.[1] It all depends on where you live, your ability to communicate, and your capacity to advocate for yourself or your family. Extending coverage to the uninsured is not as impossible as it sounds. That's because we are not starting from scratch. In fact, we are providing considerable tax funds, through Medicare, Medicaid, veterans funds, government plans, and disability payments, albeit in a highly reactive, after-the-fact way. Rather than providing insurance more broadly to those in need, and incentivizing prevention, we reactively reimburse those who assume the responsibility of caring for a population of the disadvantaged and disempowered.

Extending coverage to those currently uninsured could be accomplished without new government funding. A Kaiser

Foundation study revealed that, "If a substantial part of the financing of care received by the uninsured is already in the public sector, then some share of these funds is potentially available for transfer to new government efforts to extend coverage to those currently uninsured. Much of the $23.6 billion in payments to hospitals ... would be a reasonable candidate for reallocation ... since hospitals would be the primary beneficiaries."[2]

How much medical care do uninsured patients use? Roughly half of what the insured use, but at the expense of later entry into the health care system and poorer outcomes. Who pays for the care? We do, after the fact, through tax-supported public funds. How much uncompensated care do people receive now? Best estimates for 2001 were approximately $35 billion. How much did federal, state, and local governments expend to cover the care of the uninsured in 2001? Best estimates are $30.6 billion, with an additional $7 to $10 billion paid to hospitals and other private sources.

The best way to ensure true health equity and justice in the United States is to redirect funding to provide to the uninsured what the rest of us have—and that's health insurance. A few years ago, the U.S. health care system received a shot across the bow from the World Health Organization. The WHO had been fast at work on a comparative study of national health systems. The study considered five standards—overall level of population health, health inequalities, overall health system responsiveness, distribution of responsiveness, and distribution of financial burden. Surprising to many U.S. leaders, our national system was ranked a dismal 37th, primarily because we scored comparatively low in distribution of resources and in distribution of financial burden.[3]

The report seemed to reveal the issue of feast or famine in U.S. health. The feast? According to a 2002 Institute of Medicine report, Americans today, compared with Americans in 1900, "are healthier, live longer, and enjoy lives that are less likely to be marked by injuries, ill health, or premature death."[4] The famine? As stated by health policy experts Stephen Isaacs and Steven Schroeder in the *New England Journal of Medicine*, "Any celebration of these victories must be tempered by the realization that these gains are not shared fairly by all members of our society."[5]

The U.S. response has been to critically explore how best to expand health insurance and to critically examine racial disparities in our health system. Yet studying racial disparities in our health system isn't quite as straightforward as it may sound because, as Isaacs and Schroeder note, "Race and class are both independently associated with health status, although it is often difficult to disentangle the individual effects of the two factors."[5]

A few simple numbers illustrate this point. Whites have a median net worth in the United States that is ten times greater than blacks.[6] While 11 percent of whites live below the poverty line, 27 percent of blacks struggle with poverty.[7] The life expectancy of blacks is seven years less than that of whites. And blacks suffer higher rates of cardiovascular disease, diabetes, hypertension, infant mortality, homicide, and a variety of cancers.[8] Are these differences due primarily to race or class?

It's clear that prejudice and discrimination, the hallmarks of racism, impact the health of minorities in America, but it is becoming increasingly obvious that low socioeconomic status, which is often a byproduct of racial discrimination, also has a significant impact on health. Looking at the number of deaths per 100,000 person-years in adult men with incomes under $10,000 per year, blacks have 21 percent more deaths than whites. This difference declines to 4 percent for those with incomes from $15,000 to $25,000. But when you turn the numbers sideways, comparing whites with incomes below $10,000 with whites with incomes of $15,000 to $25,000 per year, the lower income group has 2.4 times more deaths. A similar comparison among blacks shows 2.7 times more deaths among those with lower incomes.[5]

Besides income, other socioeconomic issues intersect

with race to profoundly alter health.[8] People without a high school diploma are three times more likely to smoke than college graduates, and they're three times less likely to exercise.[9,10] And clerical civil servants in Britain have death rates from cardiovascular disease that exceed deaths rates of their administrators by 300 percent.[11]

Income, education, and employment are relatively blunt measures. But even these measures, and their relationship to a population's health, have not traditionally been captured in U.S. health policy research efforts. The United States does not systematically collect mortality and morbidity data stratified by social class.[5] Death certificates, for example, note race, but until recently did not capture employment, income, or education level.[5]

Experts debate which of these class factors primarily impacts health. Is it education, with its associated access to better jobs, embedded values, problem-solving skills, and effect on self-esteem? Is it higher income, which allows for basic needs to be met, secures better neighborhoods and schools, and allows better access to services? Or is it employment, especially jobs that provide decent working conditions, security, health insurance, and moderate stress?

Likely, it's all of the above, playing off each other and not addressable solely through traditional health programming. But we know that some factors are associated with low socioeconomic status and poor health, such as poor nutrition, increased smoking, decreased exercise, increased stress and fear, unsafe neighborhoods with high crime levels, substandard housing, inaccessible and expensive services, environmental hazards, and poor schools.[5] So it is increasingly clear that significant investment in the short- and medium-term to address socioeconomic issues could favorably impact health and health care costs over the long term. And increasingly one of the biggest hits on those with marginal socioeconomics is an episode of illness which drives individuals and families without insurance into "medical bankruptcy."

The favorable impact of improved socioeconomic status

is likely because education, transportation, recreation, housing, and tax policy all impact health policy. Studies have shown that expanding access to care, which certainly should be done, will only impact 10 percent to 15 percent of premature deaths.[12] Most of the remaining potential benefit is embedded in the expansion of healthy behaviors within individuals, families, and communities. The keys that unlock those doors are opportunity, security, and confidence in the future. Only by opening these doors including a move toward universal, secure, and transportable health insurance coverage, will health care in the United States realize its full potential.

The United States is the only developed nation in the world that relies on businesses to provide health insurance. At its peak in 2000, employer-sponsored insurance covered nearly 67percent of non-elderly Americans.[13] But the truth is, this system is breaking down, and it probably should never have been started at all. In fact, according to Princeton health economist Uwe Reinhardt, "If we had to do it over again, no policy analyst would recommend this model."[14]

So how did we get here? A couple of events in history paved the way for employer-based health insurance in the United States. The wheels were first put in motion when, in 1932, President Franklin D. Roosevelt chose to focus on Social Security instead of universal health care. And a series of government actions—some with unintended consequences—in the decades to follow further solidified our dependence on this type of system. The bottom line is, many experts agree that our employer-based health care system evolved, not necessarily accidentally, but in what can be considered an "unplanned" way that disregarded any long-term outlook.

One key to understanding this scenario is something called the "dependency ratio." This is the ratio between the number of people who aren't working in a population versus the number of people who are. Any employer who offers pensions and benefits to its employees has to deal with the consequences of this ratio.[15] But as it turns out, employers back in the 1950s most often did not.

In the early 1930s, the country was in a desperate state. As Wilbur Cohen, who served in the Roosevelt administration, would later reflect, "Roosevelt in 1933 could have federalized or nationalized anything he wanted ... at the bottom of the depression if [he] wanted to create all national banks ... a national system of Social Security and health insurance, he could have gotten it."[14]

As I mentioned, Roosevelt chose, rather, to focus on Social Security. Why he dropped health is debated. One theory points to the fierce opposition of the American Medical Association at the time. Another places the spotlight on famous neurosurgeon Harvey Cushing, Roosevelt's son's father-in-law, who had lunch with him the day before his announced decision. Whatever the reason, health insurance on a national scale was abandoned.[14]

Into the resultant void came non-profit Blue Cross and Blue Shield plans. For-profit companies watched from a distance through the 1930s. Once profitability was clear, they streamed in behind the Blues, so that by the time the country was prepared for post-World War II expansion, private insurance infrastructure was in place. It had a little help along the way. In the early years of the war, the economy super-heated and caps were placed on employee salaries to prevent inflation. Employers, competing for scarce workers, began to layer on benefits, including health insurance. By 1949, the government ruled that benefits were part of the negotiated wage package; and five years later, the IRS exempted employer-provided health benefits from income tax.[16]

Coincident with this, labor and management dueled over the issue. In 1949, the United Auto Workers Toledo local began a drive to create a regional pension plan that would spread risk across many auto industry suppliers. The reasoning was that even if your particular company went bankrupt, your benefits would be safe because they came from a regional pool, not directly from your employer. Business owners and large employers disagreed with the concept. They felt that collectivization threatened the free market and business owners' autonomy. In the United States a year later, Charlie Wilson, then president of General Motors, began offering GM workers health care benefits and a pension. The offer was more defensive than beneficent. Before this decision, Wilson had been in contract talks with Walter Reuther, the national president of the UAW. Reuther disagreed with Wilson's move, but it didn't really matter. In the single decade between 1940 and 1950, the number of Americans covered by employer-sponsored health care increased from 20 million to 142 million. Today, the number, in decline since the year 2000, stands at 159 million, which is 62.5 percent of our non-elderly population.[14]

In the decades following these events, it has become obvious to both employer and employee alike that tying one's health insurance to one's employment is problematic. For the employee, the insurance is not portable and this means that losing your job is a double hit—loss of income and loss of health insurance. For employers, careful introspection has come at a more gradual pace. Lee Iacocca in the 1980s, pleading Chrysler's case for a government bailout, was the first to identify a dollar figure subtracted from each automobile's profits based on health care.[17] Today, of course, it's more obvious. Financier Wilbur Ross says it this way: "Every country against which we compete has universal health care. That means we probably face a 15 percent cost disadvantage versus foreigners for no other reason than historical accident ... the randomness of our system is just not going to work."[15]

Part of the reason why this system is not going to work much longer has to do with the unintended consequences of several government actions. First, in 1974, the Employee Retirement Income Security Act (ERISA) was enacted to protect employees against abuses of their pension funds. As a secondary effect, it conferred certain benefits to employers who self-insured—that is, they acted as an insurance company for their own employees.[6] By doing so, they were exempted from state regulations that might, for example, impose universal coverage within state borders or demand coverage of services like in-vitro fertilization or mental health support. In addition, larger employers were able to remove and cover their healthy and wealthy workers, artificially skewing the case mix of those covered by private insurers, causing rates to go up.[14, 18]

Secondly, changes in federal accounting rules in 1990 and in 2005 forced companies to reflect long-term liabilities on their balance sheet and predict total pension and health benefit costs into the future. The shock of what this will actually cost—a shock that was reinforced by Wall Street and bond raters—caused employers to more aggressively explore strategies to eliminate long-term coverage and shift financial risk to their employees.[19, 20, 21]

In 2005, an average family coverage premium reached $10,000 per year, the annual wages for one minimum wage worker.[14] This is incredible, but cost of health care for current workers doesn't even begin to expose the size and scope of the problem. Lack of innovation or mismanagement on the part of companies can't be blamed either. The real culprit is the dependency ratio—which as I mentioned before is the relation between the number of people working in a population and the number who aren't—and its tie to the employer-based insurance approach. This is actually what has brought some of our largest, most revered U.S. companies to their knees.

GM is the perfect example. Today, it has an estimated $62 billion in health care liabilities and is under-funded for its long-term commitments to the tune of some $50 billion dollars. In 1962, the company had 464,000 U.S. employees and 40,000 retired beneficiaries. That's a dependency ratio of 1 to 12, which is 12 employees contributing to the pension of each retiree. In 2005, GM had 140,000 workers and 453,000 retirees. That's one-third of a worker to support each current retiree. Add to this the impact of layoffs and downsizing, which tends to preserve older workers, decrease workforce, and increase the number of pension-dependent retirees, and you can see why GM is in this dire situation.[15]

All of this is to say that while American business has avoided the perceived risks of regional planning and collectivization, with theoretical advantages for business autonomy and free trade, clearly, they have paid a very dear price. Today, innovations that increase efficiency and quality also increase the dependency ratio. Today, our most successful corporations are many billions of dollars behind in their health care obligations. Our corporate leaders are declaring bankruptcy to escape their own employees and to abandon the social contracts that they voluntarily embraced.

The reality is—in a global environment where business survival is a function of rapid innovation, age-independent knowledge management, real-time adjustments in role delineation, and rapidly changing value propositions, providing health insurance to an increasingly privileged few is an enormous distraction. GM's Charlie Wilson got the whole thing wrong. For markets, especially global markets, to function optimally, benefits and risks, most especially when it comes to health, must be broadly shared.

14.

Investing Wisely in Health

The voices of CEOs of large U.S. corporations can be heard around the country saying health care costs have placed them at a competitive disadvantage. This hardly seems like news considering we've seen near identical headlines for the past quarter of a century, multiple attempts to control supply and demand, and comprehensive restructuring plans like the Clinton health care bill, supported by leaders like Chrysler's Lee Iacocca—all come and go.[1]

But now the volume is getting louder and the message is becoming more urgent as global competition and aging are accelerating side by side and colliding. The bottom line is that U.S. employers—in both the public and the private sectors, from the largest to the smallest—are struggling to cope with health care costs, and the inefficiency and lost focus of our health care system are taking the well-deserved blame.

The most recent and visible expressions of CEO angst are coming from the U.S. auto industry, more specifically General Motors, in near-bankrupt status, and Ford, forced into major employee layoffs.[2,3] GM's Rick Wagoner is not happy and doesn't mince words. With 325,000 employees worldwide, GM spent $5.6 billion dollars in 2006 for the health insurance coverage of some 750,000 U.S. employees and retirees and their spouses and family members. In 2003, Ford spent $3.2 billion for coverage of 560,000 people.

Citing low U.S. global health rankings, Wagoner says, "The worst part of all this is that these very high costs don't necessarily buy the best health."[4]

Perhaps Wagoner wouldn't be so upset if GM still owned 46 percent of the U.S. auto market, as it did in 1979. It doesn't. At last count, GM had a 25 percent market share and more and more of its 9 million vehicles each year are produced overseas where workers' health care costs to the company, say, for example, in Canada, are about $120 for each car built, compared with $1,500 per car in the United States.[4] What makes it even more galling is that other business leaders like Richard Nesbitt, president of the Toronto Stock Exchange, in visits to places like the esteemed Harvard Club in New York City, have been urging U.S. investors "to pump their money into an economy where health care serves rather than shackles manufacturers." Adding fuel to the fire, Nesbitt's speech writer offers his critique saying: "It's just not clear what the advantages are in maintaining a system where about 20 percent of costs represent profits for private managers."[4]

Now, to some extent, we've heard all this before, and of course there is an opposing argument like, "Fine for you Canadians to say, as your citizens cross our borders to solve your health care access problem. And, by the way, what's all this talk about revamping your system if it's so great?" So I suppose if nothing else was going on, this could be pretty much ignored for another quarter century. But that's not the case because the problem is coming home to a city near you.

Take Duluth, Minnesota, for example. Back in 1983 they made what looked like a good deal with their city employees. It seems the employees were saving up sick time and vacation time, which rolled over year to year, and cashing it in with retirement, and this was costing the city a fortune. So, in negotiations, the city fathers cut a deal. You give up the banked time, and we'll cover your health care costs in retirement. It sounded good in 1983, but when an actuary totaled the projected costs for existing retirees and their families in

2002, it came to a staggering $178 million dollars, twice the city's annual operating budget. To add salt to their wounds, when they re-checked the figures in 2005, it had escalated to $280 million.[5]

Now what's even more interesting is what caused the city of Duluth to check in the first place. Enter GASB 45, or more correctly, Governmental Accounting Standards Board Statement #45, a new rule set to take effect on June 1, 2007.[6] Under the new rule, all states, large cities, and counties in the United States must define their 30-year liability for promised benefits to retirees and the theoretical plans in place to cover the costs. You don't, by law, have to fund the cost, but if you don't, rating agencies will likely downgrade your bonds—not a good thing if you are the city or state manager borrowing capital to keep the enterprise afloat. Agencies like Standard & Poor's have already instituted systems that assess governmental "post-employment obligations" as part of their ratings.[7]

Is Duluth an outlier? Not at all. Of the 50 states, only 11 have pre-funded retirees' benefits.[5] Most states simply have a "pay as you go" policy. The problem is, predicting what the future will look like is not so easy. It's affected by your benefit package, the future population demographics and their health status, your fund investments, and the cost of U.S. health care 30 years from now.

Well-known human resource expert Mercer estimates the total state, city, and county liability for the current 5.5 million U.S government retirees and their families to be in excess of $1 trillion.[5,8] For Ohio, things don't look so bad. They've been withdrawing 4 percent from employees' paychecks for some time and have more than $12 billion in their retirement trust fund. But for Maryland or Michigan, the future is not so bright. Neither is pre-funded, and Maryland's bill for current state employees is estimated at more than $20 billion while Michigan's tops $30 billion.[5]

When corporations like automobile manufacturers complained that paying for health care drove up their costs and decreased the global competitiveness of their products, Americans were generally unimpressed. They chose instead to focus on the general profitability of these organizations and adjusted their preferences to non-U.S. automobiles, for example, which, after all, were a better buy—one of the positive spoils of globalization. They did not see a bankrupt GM in their future, driven in part by huge under-funded promises to retirees. And even if they had, that was the GM workers' problem, not their own. But now, the virus has spread to their communities, and will affect the lives of teachers, policemen, firemen, sanitation workers, bus drivers, public health workers and others. And there is no easy fix. Even more taxes and fewer services will not be enough to bridge gaps this large.

There's an old saying, "one man's waste is another man's job." But GASB 45 has or will soon reveal that health care waste and our inability to structure the system more efficiently around prevention and wellness are now undermining job security and retirement security for a great many citizens. We are rapidly descending into the scary world of medical insolvency. And that descent is increasingly enveloping not just corporations or governments, but all of us as well.

In the United States in 2005, legislation was enacted to revamp the nation's bankruptcy laws.[4] The feeling was that citizens were finding it too easy to pursue this avenue to excuse their debt, and that in an "ownership society," rights needed to be more tightly linked to responsibility.[4] Even a cursory look at the numbers reveals why legislators were concerned. Between 1980 and 2001, there was a 360 percent increase in bankruptcy filings. In 2001, approximately 1.5 million families filed for protection that would cover 3.9 million family members, including 1.3 million children.[9]

But perhaps the sadder story here is why so many people are filing for bankruptcy and what role illness and medical bills are playing in their decision. The truth is, medical problems contribute to about half of all bankruptcies, and you'd be surprised at all the people, like those with health insurance, who think they're protected but actually are not.

The typical bankruptcy filer does not generally fit the stereotype of a chronically poor family member out of control. The reality is that the nation's poorest poor have few assets to protect and few resources to support legal costs. The average bankruptcy filer actually is around 40, possesses some college education, is slightly more likely to be female than male, is middle or working class, and owns a home. [3]

Declaring bankruptcy involves filing a petition in federal court for protection from one's creditors under the rules of bankruptcy law. By giving the court control over certain assets, all collection efforts against a debtor abruptly come to a halt. There are two avenues a debtor can take. Seventy percent choose Chapter 7, which involves liquidating all non-exempt assets. You are allowed to keep tools, clothes, and some equity in your home. But the reality for 96 percent of Chapter 7 filers is that by the time they get to this point, all assets are already gone. At the end, the debtor starts anew, free of debt, but likely not free of problems because the filings are public, which can affect future employment efforts and impact long-term credit reports and rates offered on loans for decades into the future.[9]

Thirty percent of filers choose Chapter 13, which involves a court-administered five-year negotiated payment plan. As long as you make your payments, you retain your property. Whether it's Chapter 7 or Chapter 13, you still must pay your taxes, student loans, alimony, child support, and secured loans like home mortgages if you want to hold on to your property. [9]

We've known for many years that health status and bankruptcy have been joined at the hip. Back in 1972, Senator Ted Kennedy laid this out in detail in his book, *In Critical Condition: The Crisis in America's Health Care.*[10] The facts haven't changed for the better since then. Roughly one-sixth of the U.S. population spends more than 5 percent of their disposable income on health care.[11] Approximately one-fifth at one point or another have been contacted by collection agencies related to their medical bills.[12] And if you or a family member is unlucky enough to contract a terminal illness, there is a four in ten chance of a severe financial crisis in your future.[13]

An examination of more than 1,700 U.S. debtors who declared bankruptcy in 2001 showed obvious examples of the gradual, downward, often health-related financial slide they experienced in the two years prior to filing. Out of the debtors with health issues, 38 percent had a lapse in insurance in the two-year lead up. Sixty percent avoided a necessary visit to the doctor or dentist, and 47 percent did not fill a prescription they had been given.[9]

Looking at the entire group, 28 percent cited illness or injury as their specific cause of bankruptcy. But nearly half (46 percent) met at least one of the four criteria for "major medical bankruptcy." The criteria include illness or injury as a direct cause of insolvency, uncovered medical bills exceeding $1,000, two weeks of work lost to illness or injury, or a history of mortgaging the home to pay medical bills.[9]

For that 28 percent whose illness drove them toward bankruptcy, who was sick in the family? Eight out of ten times it was the parent. In these cases there was usually a double financial hit—lost wages accounting for 65 percent of the financial loss and unplanned medical bills accounting for 35 percent of the loss. In 13 percent of the cases, a child was ill, and in 8 percent, it was an elderly family member.[9]

As for the illnesses that lead to medical bankruptcy in these families, the most common diagnoses include cardiovascular disease; trauma, orthopedic and back problems; and cancer, diabetes, pulmonary disease, psychiatric disorders, and childbirth-related and congenital disorders. The costs of childbirth and death occurred often enough to tip the scale.[9]

Surprisingly, most of those who eventually slid into medical insolvency were initially insured. More than 75 percent had coverage prior to their illness or injury. In 60 percent of the cases, the coverage was private, with one-third losing the coverage when they stopped working due to illness. Fifty-six percent could no longer afford insurance premiums, and 7 percent couldn't get new insurance due to preexisting medical conditions. On average for all of the debtors citing medical reasons for bankruptcy, the mean out-of-pocket expenditures from time of illness to bankruptcy were a surprisingly low $11,854.[9] This last figure should give pause to the current enthusiasts of Consumer-Directed Health Plans in as much as these plans offer high deductibles and steeply tiered benefits with catastrophic coverage kicking in too late to avoid financial disaster.

The truth of the matter is that if you are a working American, low or middle class, without significant savings and disability insurance, and you fall prey to a common illness that prevents you from drawing a salary, unpaid medical bills approaching the $10,000 threshold will likely cause you to consider bankruptcy to keep a roof over your family's head. Such vulnerability, along with our 45 million citizens who are completely uninsured, fundamentally undermines societal values and the theoretical framework of the "ownership society." A home-centered preventive health care system requires a stable "home." And increasingly, the insecurity inherent in our non-universal, non-transportable, and unreliable health insurance system precludes the level of economic stability necessary to plan our collective healthy futures.

15.

Managing End-of-Life Care

Decision-making at the end of life is a critical challenge for the patients, families, and physicians involved.[1] In the not-too-distant past, families and physicians were often complicit in hiding information from terminally ill patients. Studies show that this practice is much less frequent today. However, physicians in a 2001 study were found to understate the severity of a terminally ill patient's prognosis 63 percent of the time, and there is general agreement that physicians and health institutions continue to overuse technology and under-use communication when dealing with terminally ill patients.[2] To reinforce this point, an examination of hospital records of 164 patients with significant dementia and terminal metastatic cancer showed that nearly half of the patients received aggressive non-palliative treatments and a quarter received cardiopulmonary resuscitation.[3]

While it's easy in retrospect to critique such behaviors, the reality is that managing the progression toward death is highly complex. The physician is often asked to bridge the chasm between life-saving and life-enhancing care. Guidance must be highly personalized and must consider prognosis, the risks and benefits of various interventions, the patient's symptom burden, the timeline ahead, the age and stage of life of the patient, and the quality of the patient's support system.

Considering all these, the physician, patient, and family are expected to explore all curative options, provide clear and honest communications, invite family input, provide their best recommendations, and ultimately affirm and support a patient's decision.[1]

Walking the road of terminal illness carries special burdens for all involved. For the patient and family, shock gives way to a complex analysis that often intersects with guilt, regret, and anger. Fear must be managed and channeled, and loss and its implications for family and loved ones cannot be avoided. On top of this, there are multiple complex decisions that must be addressed within specific time constraints.

While all this is extremely difficult for patients and families, it's also demanding of physicians.[4,5] The sheer complexity of individualizing and humanizing each passage is complicated by a heavy emotional burden that comes with accepting responsibility for the care of others. Physicians struggle to balance hopefulness with truthfulness. Determining "how much information," "within what space of time," and "with what degree of directness for this particular patient" requires a skillful commitment that matures with age and experience.

Managing both physical and mental health and distinguishing between normal grief and clinical depression add to the challenge.

Finally, incorporating the unique culture and spiritual context that can help define the right course of action for each individual demands a special set of eyes and ears and an ability to reach out and touch.

Studies confirm that 85 percent of terminally ill patients desire as much information as they can get, good or bad. Prognostic information is the most important. Only 7 percent of terminally ill patients seek "good news" exclusively and only 8 percent want no details.[4,5]

When a diagnosis is first made, everyone's focus is on life preservation. But a sharp decline, results of diagnostic studies, or an internal awareness can signal a transition and lead patients and families to recognize that death is approaching. Once acceptance arrives, end-of-life decision-making naturally follows. Denying that death is approaching only compresses the timeline for these decisions, adds anxiety, and undermines the sense of control over one's own destiny.

With acceptance, the goals become quality of life and comfort. Physicians, hospice, family, and other caregivers can focus on assessing physical symptoms, psychological and spiritual needs, quality of support systems, estimation of prognosis, and defining a patient's end-of-life goals.[2] How important might it be for a patient to attend a granddaughter's wedding or see one last Christmas, and are these realistic goals to pursue?

One issue that often gets confused in the process of planning a death with dignity is hope. It is possible to die with hope, with self-control, and with dignity, but it requires some time and planning. Physician participation is critical. End-of-life care expert Dr. David Weissman offers this counsel: "Physicians are often reluctant to provide specific information largely out of fear of destroying hope.... Dying patients can still have hope for system control, for resolving personal relationships, and for a dignified death."[1]

In order to plan a death with dignity, we need to acknowledge death as a part of life—an experience to be embraced rather than ignored when the time comes. Recognizing when that time has arrived is a critical challenge for each of us. I recently experienced two deaths in my family. One, my 50-year-old brother-in-law, married to my younger sister, who suffered from pancreatic cancer. Together, they were the parents of three teenage children. The other, my wife's mother, who suffered from multiple chronic diseases and dementia, who died in her 90th year.

Both deaths involved the complex dynamics of a large family. I am one of 12 children and my wife is one of ten. Both loved ones died at home. Both had the assistance of Hospice. And both progressed through a series of stages that taxed the families' management and organizational skills.

Author and psychiatrist Elisabeth Kubler-Ross described the five stages of grief as denial, anger, bargaining, depression, and acceptance.[6] Roberta Temes' book, *Living with an Empty Chair*, outlines three stages: numbness, disorganization, and reorganization.[7] While both have merit, and our families encountered all eight of these stages in varying orders and in differing ways, they do not cover the more predictable organizational stages we encountered, nor do they define the management challenges associated with each stage.

So I have put together what I describe as the four organizational stages of dying: engagement, release, testimony, and recovery. The first stage, engagement, focuses on confronting the threat, exploring options for combating it, making decisions about how best to proceed, and following through on those decisions. Depending on the threat, time may or may not be an issue. For my brother-in-law, facing an aggressive cancer, time was of the essence. For my mother-in-law, with diabetes and dementia, not so much.

During engagement, the patient, family, and care team are expected to explore all curative options, provide clear and honest communications, invite family input, provide best recommendations, and ultimately affirm and support the patient's decision. This requires an organizational linkage that may be as uncomplicated as a trusted physician's office, as in my mother-in-law's case, or as complex as dealing with experimental research protocols and interdisciplinary cancer centers, as in my brother-in-law's case. In general, however, engagement translates into five management challenges. First is fact-finding through personal research and outreach and through expert opinion and advice, facilitated by the establishment of trust and confidence. Second is decision-making, directed at type and course of therapy. Third is intervention, executing the treatment plan, whether long-term or short-term. Fourth is monitoring to assess success and being able to make informed adjustments to the treatment plan. And fifth is active, ongoing reassessment with focus on risks and benefits of each decision point, and consideration not only of life but also quality of life.

The second stage is release. Having engaged and pursued reasonable steps to survive, without success, those involved have to acknowledge that death must now be accepted as a near-term reliability. For my brother-in-law, this reality set in during a third round of chemotherapy, after two previous regimens had failed, and bowel obstruction set in during the fifth of his six months of life following diagnosis. For my mother-in-law, this was a much more subtle and personal transition. She seemed to know when the time was right, almost "choosing her time," and death came ten days later.

Whether chronic or acute, young or old, when a diagnosis is first made, everyone's focus is on life preservation. But in the face of declining options, hopefulness collides with truthfulness. And the truth can be harsh and undeniable, especially for the young who haven't had as much time to mentally prepare. But for all ages, stage 2, release, requires acceptance by both patient and loved ones. Readiness varies, and for progress to occur, there must be alignment and a common vision of what is to come. The focus shifts from life preservation to life enhancement. Quality of remaining life is tied to adjustments in the physical environment (such as moving a bed to the first floor) and ensuring that pain and other symptoms, such as nausea, are effectively managed. Support must be enlisted and resources marshaled.

For my brother-in-law, this meant having one of our sisters, who is a registered nurse, move in for the last two weeks of his life, working in tandem with the family. They also involved Hospice and home visits by his physicians. For my mother-in-law, during the last week, it meant that my wife's four sisters joined her and the in-house caregiver who had managed her dementia for many years. They involved Hospice to help with pain management and provide support for their mother as they accepted the dying process.

Because of the environment, we, as the family, were organized, and because the patients were relatively pain-free but fully conscious, they were able to conduct extensive and enlightened visitations during the closing days. This prepared the families and loved ones for the future and allowed what "needed to be said" to be said. It also created a transcendent atmosphere of great spirit to mix with the seemingly unbearable sorrow and loss. Words were exchanged that we will long remember.

With death, we arrive at the third stage: testimony. How should loved ones be remembered? This is under the control of the living. The obituary, funeral arrangements, family travel, eulogy, burial, and various memorial rituals all require attention. Of the four organizational stages of death, this may be the one most routinely mismanaged. It is critically important, not only in communicating the value and meaning of one's life, and the lives he or she touched, but also in beginning the healing process, and often allowing old wounds to be repaired, and disrupted lives to begin anew. Among the management challenges, first and foremost is inclusion—involvement of as many family members and loved ones as possible. Second is planning, including finances, timing of services, and communication before, during, and after the ceremony. Third is performance—readings, eulogies, informal story-telling, photo boards, and displays of items important to the individual and the bereaved. Fourth is comforting—coming together to manage those stricken, injured, and weakened by the course of events. And the fifth management challenge is the act of memorializing, which is an opportunity to reinforce goodness, humor, and values that deserve a spotlight. By memorializing, we challenge ourselves to live a better and more complete life.

The final organizational stage of dying is recovery—assisting loved ones in absorbing the loss and remembering in a way that advances the physical, mental, and spiritual health of the bereaved.[8] There is not a perfect path or consistent timetable, but the management challenges associated with recovery are somewhat predictable. They include managing shock, confusion, and disorientation; accepting the loss; sustaining individual self-worth; pacing recovery; identifying complicated grief if it persists and seeking professional help if it's needed; and, finally, reinvesting in relationships.

Each of these four stages of the dying process have common elements. But each is a unique management challenge in its own right. Similarities include that each stage is complex, requires planning, demands decisions, causes fatigue, and requires team support. But, true success comes with the insight that each of the four stages is fundamentally different—they involve different missions, players, organizational interfaces, support staff, time pressures, and measures of success.

16.
The Best
Place to Die

As baby boomers in the United States move en masse toward seniordom, they are beginning to focus as much on dying well as living well. It's not that they are morbid. It's that many of them are seeing the vision of the future in their own parents' reflections.

Twenty-five percent of American households now have family caregivers, mostly women and mostly boomers.[1] And it's the nature of the generation to ramp up expectations and to rebuild them to higher specifications. Currently, they don't like what they see, especially in an age where health care partnerships are replacing paternalism, and health consumers are devouring empowering educational information.[2]

The health community is getting the message and has realized that defining a "good death" requires input from patients and loved ones. The patient is looking for comfort, respect, emotional support, information, and well-coordinated care. And to no one's surprise, loved ones are looking for the same things.[3]

What is today's deathbed reality? It is that nearly seven out of ten of us—some 69 percent—die in institutional settings—such as nursing homes or hospitals. More than three in ten, or 31 percent, die at home. Of those who die at home, 36 percent die without any caregiver present, 12 percent have the benefit of some nursing care, and 52 percent are supported by hospice services.[4]

The Hospice movement was begun in 1946 with St. Christopher's Hospice in England.[5] It championed a holistic approach to the care of terminally ill patients, primarily those with cancer. Over the years, the approach has been extended to a wide variety of patients with terminal illnesses, and has spread around the globe. In the United States, however, access to insurance coverage for hospice services for terminally ill seniors who do not have cancer remains problematic. It requires certification from two physicians that the patient only has six months to live. Predicting this for chronic disease can be less reliable than for cancer.[6]

The various sites in which people die are associated with different understandings of disease states, different financial circumstances, and different capacities to support the extensive needs of dying patients. They are also associated with different patient groups. For instance, elderly women who are not married are disproportionately represented among nursing home deaths.[4] But is that a problem? After all, what better place to die than in an institution with trained personnel, intravenous medications, and lots of technology?

A recent study surveying loved ones of patients who died indicates that it may be worth the effort to carefully plan where you wish to die. The satisfaction of loved ones with the care of dying family members or friends varies widely by site and staffing. Managing the symptoms of pain and shortness of breath is problematic for a patient dying at home with only some nursing help, but improves if hospice services are in place. Nursing homes show weaknesses in these areas as well, while hospitals do well at managing pain, and are the best at managing shortness of breath.[4]

In terms of emotional support and respect for the patient, Hospice care is clearly the leader. For example, the study showed that in the judgment of surviving loved ones, only 35 percent of Hospice patients lacked adequate emotional support, while 52 percent of hospital patients felt neglected. And while only 4 percent of Hospice patients felt respect for them was wanting, 20 percent of hospital patients perceived disrespect.[4]

The study also revealed differences in how the patients' loved ones were treated. Hospice once again markedly outperformed all others. Dissatisfaction with the level of family contact with physicians was only 14 percent in Hospice compared with 31 percent in nursing homes and 51 percent in hospitals. Inadequate emotional support for families and loved ones was 21 percent in Hospice compared with 36 percent in nursing homes and 38 percent in hospitals; and faulty information support for loved ones was a problem in 29 percent of Hospice cases, compared with 44 percent in nursing homes and 50 percent in hospitals.[4]

Overall, looking at the needs of dying patients and the needs of their families and loved ones, it's not just site, but staff, that counts. Less-than-excellent care was noted 29 percent of the time with Hospice care, compared with 58 percent of the time with nursing homes and 53 percent with hospitals. But it's not just being at home that makes the difference, because patients dying at home with just some nursing services experienced less-than-excellent care just as frequently as those in hospitals.[4]

Careful planning can make a "good death" a more likely outcome for patients and loved ones. In some cases, an institutional setting is the only appropriate choice, as with a patient in extreme pain or respiratory distress. But in general, hospitals and nursing homes appear challenged—with the conflicting demands of acute and chronic care, staffing and budget limitations, and the complexity of operations—to manage the complex and personalized needs of a dying patient and loved ones to a harmonious conclusion.

Hospice care is not perfect. For example it could improve care of shortness of breath and emotional support for patients. But the idea of holistic care comes closer to achieving the ideal of a "good death" than any of the current options.

We should build on that ideal of what is necessary for a "good death"—a supportive site, sustained multifaceted care, anticipating rather than reacting to needs. When you critically examine the needs for a "good death," a successful home-centered health system would be well-positioned to support and contribute both information and compassion for both patient and loved ones.

17.

Predictions for 2015

L et me now share with you three visions that I believe will play out within the next ten years. The first is the re-emergence of home-centered care. It has now become clear to most that nearly 100 percent of the assets we currently define as our health care system—the bricks and mortar of our hospitals and our patient offices; our human resources as embodied in our training, roles, responsibilities, and payment incentives; our educational curricula; and our continuously reengineered processes targeted at in-patient safety and efficiency—have little to offer us, in their current form, to assist the build-out of a truly preventive health care system. Rather, these elements are original, or second or third, iterations of a century-old interventional care system that stubbornly survives largely in its original form because we have been unsuccessful in managing and executing the creation of a more inclusive and anticipatory health care system.

Prevention is grounded in education and behavioral modification. It begins before birth and extends beyond death. To be successful, a preventive health care system must advantage multigenerational relationships to provide multiple, repetitive inputs in real time that allow micro-adjustments in one's daily life. Such a system demands intimately informed, highly motivated, deeply committed individuals willing to gently prod those under their charge toward health and wellness. Prevention presumes guiding hands and 24/7 presence, family and community linkages, and the ability to efficiently lay out lifecycle plans and execute lifespan management on the one hand, and ensure adherence to palliative treatment plans for patients with chronic disease on the other. All of this is 180° apart from what we have traditionally termed health care.

In centering the build-out of such a health care system, there is only one place that is both geographically identifiable and politically viable as a candidate. That is the home. And while homes vary widely, from cardboard containers constructed hastily to shield the rain to "McMansions" that consume more than they provide, homes of all varieties share a special place in our hearts.

But while home may be where the heart is, it is most certainly not currently where the health is. That could change. GE recognized the "moldability" of the home when it launched its remarkable exhibit called the "Carousel of Progress" at the World Fair in New York in 1964. As a 16-year-old, I remember sitting in the revolving theatre and witnessing the six decades peel away with the last look peering 20 years into the future. At the end, I had to admit that, in improving our toasters and refrigerators, GE had truly improved our lives.

It is fair to imagine, then, that the same could be done with health. And just as we in America view homelessness as a social failure, we have begun to view healthlessness in the same light. If we were able to equitably re-outfit and at least partially improve the health of homes by leveraging technology—informational technology, diagnostic and imaging technology, entertainment technology, financial system technology—could we efficiently re-center our health care system around the home? As it turns out, others have been asking this same question and have been actively at work, below the radar screen, developing a wide range of product offerings that Forrester Research forecasts will find an explosive growth market beginning in 2010 and becoming fully robust by 2015. Literally thousands of technology, entertainment, and financial firms are now investing in the parallel build-out of preventive home-centered health. And in this effort they are working side by side with governments and municipalities, and with major academic engineering powerhouses such as MIT, the University of Rochester, Carnegie Mellon, and the University of Michigan. What is surprising, however, is the relative absence of the patient-physician relationship, care teams, and multigenerational prevention in the home health planning visions of these groups. Rather, the emphasis has been on the use of consumer health electronics to support independence, aging in place at home, and chronic disease management, when the true opportunity lies in multigenerational lifecycle management.

In 2005, in partnership with leaders from Intel and the American Association of Homes and Services for the Aging (AASHA), a new and fuller vision emerged. At the center of this vision is the home. The primary health information loop would not be from hospital to physician's office and back, but rather from home to care team and back to home. Informal caregivers would become fully enfranchised members of physician-led, often nurse-directed care teams. These family caregivers would not only be linked virtually to their multigenerational families and to their care teams, but also to other informal family caregivers—effectively addressing the profound sense of isolation that comes with these roles. A wide range of secondary loops would evolve from generalist to specialist, from clinician's office to hospital, from care team to insurer or pharmacy. But the primary loop, where data would originate and from which privacy access would be granted, would be home-centered.

The data flowing out of the home would be rich, varied, real-time, and virtual. It would include vital signs and diagnostic and imaging results sent wirelessly to care teams. But beyond this, the healthy home would have pervasive, low-cost sensors able to track motions, actions, and interactions. Data emanating from these sensors would be interpreted by on-site intelligence software and measured against predicted healthy living plans. The results would be fed in a continuous stream to the care team. Coming the other way, in the feedback loop, supported by a 24/7 connecting interface, would be a human team partner communicating through a friendly interface of your choice—wristwatch, phone, radio, TV, or computer—a guide and companion who might remind you to bathe if you've forgotten; to increase fluid, alter diet, or exercise; to take your meds or vary your dose today; or to call your daughter as you had promised.

Physician-led teams would be reimbursed for managing complexity. Informal caregivers would become home health managers, rewarded with lower health insurance premiums or tax benefits for accomplishing healthy family outcomes. Nurses' roles as coaches, educators, and behavior modifiers would expand with the full support and encouragement of physicians. Offices would see much less traffic, as most care could be accomplished without a visit. Yet physicians would make a good living, and even have time to visit their patients, from time to time, in their own homes.

The second vision, flowing once again from our five intersecting megatrends, I call "collapsing databases." Three enormous health databases are in the process of going virtual or electronic. The first of these is the Clinical Research Database or CRD. On the back end of the Vioxx withdrawal, conflict-of-interest concerns, and legitimate health consumer desires for early access to discovery information, major research databases are moving toward open transparency. For better or worse, the public will soon have ready electronic access to the vast majority of positive and negative results of studies at the time of completion. These results will be virtual and readily transferable, far and wide.

The second database is the Continuing Medical Education or CME database. It, too, is going electronic. In fact, nearly 20 percent of all U.S. CME is already electronic and has been demonstrated to be effective. It is likely that within ten years, the vast majority of CME will be virtual and will be applied in real time rather than in episodic segments. Hand-held devices are increasingly standard medical equipment in caring encounters, providing immediate database support to the patient-physician relationship during the evaluative and joint decision-making process. This allows experts to quite confidently predict that in a preventive health care system, where information is overwhelmingly the dominant health care product, CME will be interchangeable and indecipherable from the care itself.

And this brings us to the third database, one I call CCE or Continuing Consumer Education. As the consumer health movement continues to evolve from educational empowerment to active engagement and inclusion in the health care team, patients and their families will demand access to the same hand-held mobile hardware and information software that the other care team members are using. This will help avoid any confusion that might arise from multi-tracked information and accelerate the need for simple and well-designed educational products. By using the same devices and mobile educational platforms, issues of varying e-standards and problems of incompatibility that might compromise the primary "home to care team to home" loop will melt away.

So these three large, growing databases—CRD, CME, CCE—have gone virtual and are widely accessible. What remains are two translation gaps. The first is between CRD and CME, and it ensures that discoveries will take many years to penetrate and inform clinical practice. If, for example, a study reveals that it is safer and better for mother and child to provide epidural anesthesia at 2 cm rather than 5 cm dilation during labor, and that doing so not only does not increase C-section rates but ensures safer, more comfortable labor and better Apgar scores for the baby, under our current system, this knowledge transfer to practice is a multiyear affair. But with virtual CRD and CME, there exists the ability to collapse those databases upon each other and almost immediately affect practice behavior changes to the benefit of thousands of current mothers and newborns coincident with this new discovery.

If CRD and CME will collapse upon each other, CME and CCE will in many ways become one and the same. Here again we are challenged by a translation gap, a gap between clinical practice (and the recommendations that flow from health professionals) and adherence to agreed-upon plans by the patients themselves. Currently patients adhere to plans at best only 50 percent of the time. The people need to be fully integrated with the people caring for the people. Thus, the frantic efforts to develop personal health records on the one hand and electronic medical records on the other are already raising entrepreneurial eyebrows. Are these not, after all, one and the same? Does not all clinical data originate with the people? Do the people not loan this data to the people in whom they have the greatest trust and confidence—their physicians, nurses, and other caregivers? And if our records are one and the same, should we not also use the same informational resources to support our joint decision making? Wouldn't this be the best way to help us stay on the same page and avoid any chance of miscalculation, misinformation, or mistake?

So the second vision is that, as we move from intervention to prevention, health care will be an information, decision, and planning dominated product or service, and this product will be anchored by three massive, collapsing databases—discovery (CRD), medical (CME), and consumer (CCE)—with primary ownership residing where the data originated, with the people, and provided primarily to the people caring for the people.

The third and final vision I call "Silo Vaporization."

Rigid silos are not unique to health care, but in health care they have been raised to an art form. Silo rigidity is a function of strongly held ideological positions or policies reinforcing backward-facing command and control systems. Fear of territorial intrusion, fear of erosion of financial resources, relatively fixed at 16 percent of our Gross National Product, and fear of change have created ideal conditions for maintenance of the status quo. Let there be no mistake about it. Our disorganized and disintegrated health care system continues to exist today because the powers on all sides of health care have felt that organizing a more rational and cogent national approach would carry with it price compression, limits in access, and loss of control. But in preserving this broken system we have supported such massive inefficiency, cost escalation, and flawed systems and processes, that what we were trying to prevent has occurred anyway. The bottom line? We are now experiencing market-induced cost compression and service and quality disintegration on a massive scale.

The ever-advancing megatrends will continue to stress and disrupt our status-quo. Eventually, our silos will vaporize completely. Let me explain how, starting with several recent developments that have quietly altered the health care landscape:

- Just four years ago, UnitedHealth Care purchased the first insurer-owned bank. Late last year, BlueCross BlueShield announced its own Blue Healthcare Bank, giving its members a place to save and withdraw money for health expenses.

- In 2005, roughly 300 of the world's largest banks and financial institutions entered the health care service sector because they saw a unique opportunity for profitability in the form of Health Savings Accounts.

- In 2006, 150 additional entrants joined the Health Savings Account bandwagon, seeking out the opportunity to leverage their vast information technology, investment expertise, and system management skills to simultaneously manage an investment portfolio of $75 billion while managing millions of daily transaction points off a health debit card, each with a fee.

- And over the space of the last several years, 400 of the largest multinational electronic, computer, and media firms, seeing the future of prevention, joined together in a single national advocacy organization called the Center for Aging Services Technologies in Washington D.C., with long-term care industry providers and the prevention and wellness community working together to drive health into the home, with or without a care team.

Now let's fast-forward eight years.

It's 2015. The national medical organizations and the national nursing organizations are locked in place. They have successfully check and check-mated each other on the issue of who writes the prescription, an important issue since the prescription has meant a visit, and the visit has always meant a fee.

The ideological face-off has generated enough heat and fear on both sides to reinforce their backward facing silos and has so preoccupied them as to prevent either from noticing the changes all around them. Yet they opened the doors of health care a decade earlier to new industries—financial institutions, technology firms, entrepreneurs—that knew how to build-out something brand new, and were not burdened by a century of ideological baggage.

So it's 2015, and nursing and medicine stand face to face, engaged, puffed up, pens drawn, ready to write the best prescription. But there are very few prescriptions left to write. Prescriptions have given way to lifecycle health planning, where adherence management has automated long-term therapies and consumer coaching has transferred many of the decisions. Most of the health databases are now merged, and a new health care system has appeared.

The people are still there, but the people who care for

the people—who processed their fears and worries, who reinforced their ties to family and community, who pointed them toward a hopeful future—are strangely absent. You see, they were not part of the build-out. For nursing and medicine, the battle is over. The reason for the battle and the reason for the silos are no longer relevant. They have awakened in 2015 and POOF! Their silos have vaporized into thin air, overtaken by a new reality created and driven by new entrants.

This is what could happen, not what must happen. The alternative to vaporization is constructive transformation. And that's still possible. Much is at stake, and it's essential to have the people and the people caring for the people work together on a build-out of a preventive home-centered health care system based on the concepts I discussed in this book.

So that you might not consider me delusional, please understand that I know that many of these concepts represent an idealized version of the best we might hope for in a resource-rich, affluent American home. But know, as well, that these concepts – a primary loop from home to care team to home; physician-nurse partnering; informal family caregiver inclusion; automated, family-centered data outflow; 24/7 assessment and coaching feedback; advanced medical communications with elimination of discovery to clinician to patient translation gaps; and active targeting of our most vulnerable populations, whether they be elderly in Florida, rural in Montana, or poor and disabled in Tucson or West Philadelphia—are both sound and achievable if we are willing to serve and if we are willing to lead.

Make no mistake: The trends that I have shared with you today will continue to accelerate us toward a home-centered health care vision—with or without physicians, nurses, and care-givers. The point is that, without us, the vision can never be truly complete. Absent mutual advocacy without the active voice of physicians at the forefront, consumerism points toward an entirely different and more hollow set of end points. Knowledge will still rise. Financial, technology, and entertainment vendors will still succeed in the creation, marketing, and sales of products that transform our homes. But relationships will fall away, and along with them the confidence and trust in each other to pursue the best for health.

Under these circumstances, our double-connect to each other becomes a double-check on each other. The bright promise of health populism reverts to the dead weight of health siloism, an outmoded concept that serves no one.

In closing, let me share with you the ten rules of health populism, as I believe they must guide and instruct our future actions:

1. When confronting a new opportunity, ask two questions, in this order:
    a. Is this good for the people and the people caring for the people?
    b. Is this good for the organization? If the answer to the first question is "no," don't ask the second question.

2. Never pursue a strategy, even if short-term and profitable, if it undermines the people's relationships with their caregivers.

3. When "building-out," build to the future and not the present.

4. The 90/10 rule: When seeking allies, embrace those with whom you share 90 percent value alignment. Have the discipline to embrace the 90 percent that connects you, and the prudence to avoid triggering the 10 percent that separates you.

5. Behave more like an NGO and less like a professional, educational, government, or business association.

6. Be transparent. Never speak through radical ideologues. Speak for yourself.

7. Stick up for the people. Make informal caregivers part of your health care team.

8. Embrace new media and circle back to traditional media. Education is the business of caregivers and the core of prevention.

9. Advocate that the primary health information highway go from home to care team to home. Links from hospital to office are secondary, not primary, links.

10. Get into the home. Get into the world.

The home is where the heart is. It must now become where the health is as well.

From Mainframe to Personal Healthcare, with Urgency

ERIC DISHMAN

O ur nation—indeed, most of our planet—faces disruptive demographic shifts that will change not only the faces of those around us in the grocery store, but also the very notions of what it means to be "old", "healthy", "sick", and "retired". As Mike Magee foretells, with cautionary optimism and passionate vision, this age wave will also transform our healthcare paradigm, bringing forth a future that may need to learn from a distant past of home-centered, family-centric, community-supported care. The question is: will we prepare for—and design infrastructure for—this perfect storm of economic, cultural, and technology trends or will we ignore the forecasts only to find ourselves in emergency response mode once the storm is battering our front door?

Today's healthcare paradigm is rooted in a reactive, crisis-driven, fix-what-is-broken model that requires and relies upon an often expensive, urban megaplex of healthcare experts and equipment. As with mainframe computers only a couple of decades ago, today we have to make a pilgrimage to that hospital mainframe to wait ever so patiently as we time-share those miraculous modern medical capabilities that have been gathered there. In the midst of already ballooning healthcare costs, growing ranks of un- and under-insured, and epidemics of age-related illnesses and injuries, this mainframe model cannot scale to meet the needs of our aging population where neither the dollars nor the doctors will exist to deliver healthcare business as usual.

Just as we moved from mainframe to personal computers that are now part of our everyday lives at home, work, and play, so, too, we must redistribute healthcare expertise and equipment from mainframe megaplexes to our homes and to our personal lives. And just as it was difficult for most of us to imagine and anticipate the changes that the PC and the Internet would bring about in society, so, too, is it difficult to conceptualize how healthcare should be transformed. Magee's vision—built upon his astute analysis of the megatrends of aging, consumerism, new patient/physician relationships, the Internet, and the rise of NGOs—offers us a glimpse, if not a roadmap, of where we must go.

Over the past 8 years, I have had the privilege to work with Intel's social science team who have interviewed, observed, and lived with over 1000 families in more than 20 countries where we have heard two common refrains: "give me systems that help me deal with my chronic disease" and, even more urgently, "give me technologies that help my parents to grow old gracefully from their own home." It is clear that the next generation of seniors will have different expectations and capacities for living the third age of their lives than have previous generations. An emphasis on home—not only the physical place that people prefer to live, but also the comfort of familiar routines and community support that come with it—is imperative if we are to insure a better and affordable quality of life for large segments of the population who will live well into their 90s, even 100s.

So how do we begin to move from the mainframe, hospital-centric model to the personal, home-centric model? What are we to do to prepare for the storm? Listing the recipe may be far easier than cooking the gourmet meal, but I believe these are some key steps to enabling Magee's vision:

1. **Admit that we have a problem.**
   Far too few politicians, providers, and consum-

ers are willing and able to discuss the impending healthcare crisis that is coming as a result of the age wave. We must find some middle ground discourse—somewhere between the gloom-and-doom approach and the head-in-the-sand approach, somewhere between dystopia and utopia—that enables an international conversation about the age wave and how we should prepare for it.

2. **Evangelize a different vision of where we need to go.**
The pages before us from Magee offer key elements of an international vision of "what's needed?" and "what's next?" in healthcare. Whether it is called "home centered care" or "personal health" or any other phrase, we have to posit a direction to move in and start the journey with a willingness to redirect as needed. Magee's metaphor of the "carousel of progress" is apt. No single vision captures everything; no single vision wins. But a carousel of related visions—rotating in front of our collective imaginations with variations on a theme—will at the very least help us decide as a nation what we aspire to be and where we want to go with healthcare.

3. **Build coalitions of like-minded organizations, companies, associations, & individuals.**
No one organization or entity can marshal the reservoir of political will and capital that will be required to unhinge our old healthcare paradigm to make way for a new one. I have worked with Larry Minnix of AAHSA and Mike Magee from Health Politics and dozens of others to create CAST, the Center for Aging Services Technologies (www.agintech.org) as one small attempt to band together hundreds of universities, technol-

ogy innovators, companies, government leaders, and providers to advocate for explicit innovation to prepare for the age wave. CAST is not the answer, either; it will take coalitions of coalitions like CAST to push for the paradigm change that is urgently required.

4. **Understand the needs of the whole care network.**
   Too often, we design healthcare systems with only one particular constituent in mind—making the doctor more efficient or empowering the patient with more knowledge about his or her disease. But we have to understand—through anthropological and sociological methods—all of the actors who make up the caregiver network, across the care continuum of care, and around the world. The trinity of patient-provider-family must be our unit of analysis and innovation.

5. **Target specific problems with technology innovation.**
   We have a tendency in modern society to just "throw" technology into the mix without having a clear set of prioritized problems that we are using technology to solve. In our work at Intel, for example, we have some specific design goals around aging—"developing technologies to prevent the majority of falls from ever happening" or "inventing systems that help reduce social isolation and loneliness for seniors"—that become the rallying cries and focus areas for our investment and innovation. Home-centered health care demands a problem-focused approach to technology innovation.

6. **Build evidence-based bodies of knowledge and evidence.**
   The move towards home-centric care cannot

happen on a whim or on untested technologies. We must use an evidence-based approach to technology innovation, where controlled studies and comparative pilots of new technologies are deployed to help determine efficacy and ROI of these new systems. Moving today's technology pilots of personal health devices from small-scale experiments to large-scale clinical trials is critical if we are to develop a marketplace of healthy, helpful, home-centered solutions.

7. **Implement. Iterate. Implement. Iterate.**
   Iterative design of home-centered technologies is an absolute necessity. The array of personal technologies available—personal computers, cell phones, MP3 players, PDAs, video players, HDTVs—and the array of chronic conditions and injuries that one can be faced with create enormous complexity and variability. There is no escaping the need for relentless experimentation and revision to bring home health technologies to the marketplace, particularly as they will be used increasingly by older people who may struggle with cognitive and physical challenges that come later in life. We must learn by doing, and know full well that none of it will be perfect the first time out of the gate.

As I write this, I have just finished a call with my father who told me the latest healthcare news about my 98-year old grandfather, who still struggles to recover from a fall he suffered last summer. Only a few weeks after his fall, my wife's grandmother also fell, which ultimately led to her death. These personal experiences occur thousands of times a day and million of times a year to people everywhere. So the storm is already here. We need to enact Mike Magee's vision of home-centered health care with some urgency. To do so, we need the moral equivalent of the "Y2K" challenge that galvanized consumers, industries, and governments to work together to prepare and update our infrastructure to avert a major technological/financial crisis as computers clocked over to the year 2000. This time around our challenge is no less urgent, the risks even more significant, and the timing every bit as predictable. We face the "Y2K + 10" challenge, when the first Baby Boomers reach retirement eligibility in the United States at the end of this decade. With persistent vision, coalition, innovation, and iteration, we can—and certainly must—prepare for this inevitability. And as Dr. Magee calls upon us to do, we can and certainly must go home again.

Eric Dishman

General Manager,
Health Research & Innovation Group, Intel Corporation
Chair, Center for Aging Services Technologies, CAST

References

CHAPTER 1

1. Alliance for Aging Research. Medical Never-Never Land Ten Reasons Why America is Not Ready for the Coming Age Boom." February 2002.

2. National Alliance for Caregiving, AARP, MetLife. Caregiving in the U.S. April 2004. Cited in MetLife, National Alliance for Caregiving. Miles Away: The MetLife Study of Long-Distance Caregiving, July 2004.

3. Magee, M. and D'Antonio, M. *The Best Medicine*. New York. St. Martin's Press; 2000.

4. Nash, D. *Connecting with the New Health Care Consumer*. New York. McGraw Hill. 2001.

5. Cohen, JL. Human Population: The Next Half Century. *Science*. Nov. 14, 2004: 1172-1175.

6. Forrester Research. Healthcare Unbound: Early Self Pay Market. Available at: www.forrester.com/Research/Document/Script/0.7211.36802.00.html. Accessed Apr. 26, 2007

7. Flynn, LJ. Some Worries as San Francisco Goes Wireless. *The New York Times*. April 10, 2006. C5.

8. Gnatek, T. Technology: Services. *The New York Times*. May 3, 2006.

9. Dishman, E. Inventing Wellness Systems for Aging in Place. Computer. 2004; 37:34-41.

10. Center for Aging Services and Technologies. Imagine—The Future of Aging. Available at: www.agingtech.org/imagine_video.aspx. Accessed April 26, 2007

11. Morrison, RS and Meier, DE. Palliative Care. NEJM. 2004;350:2582-2590.

12. Expert Panel. AIMA. "Personal Health Records and Electronic Health Records: Navigating the Intersection." Bethesda, MD. Sept. 28-29, 2006.

13. Robinson, JC. Reinvention of health insurance in the consumer era. *JAMA*. 2004; 291:1880-1886.

CHAPTER 2

1. Brundtland, GH. Speech on burden of disease concept at Hopitaux Universitaires de Geneve: December 15, 1998.

2. Bambra, C., Fox, D., Scott-Samuel, A. Towards a Politics of Health. *Health Promotion International*. 2005;20:187-193.

3. Alliance for Aging Research. Medical Never-Never Land Ten Reasons Why America is Not Ready for the Coming Age Boom." February 2002.

4. National Center for Health Statistics. 2000.

5. Arno, PS. Levine, C. Memmott MM. The economic value of informal caregiving. *Health Affairs*. 1999; 18:182-188.

6. Schultz, R. et. al. Psychiatric and physical morbidity effects of dementia

caregiving: prevalence, correlates, and causes. *Gerontologist*. 1995; 35:771-91.

7. Magee, M. Enduring Relationships in American Society. New York: Yankelovich Partners, Omnibus Study; 1999.

8. Chan, KM et al. Exercise interventions: Defusing the world's osteoporosis time bomb. Bulletin of the World Health Organization. 2003; 81:827-830.

9. Magee, M. Relationship Based Health Care in United States, United Kingdom, Canada, Germany, South Africa, and Japan. World Medical Association. Helsinki, Finland. Sept. 11, 2003.

10. Yach, D., et al. The Global Burden of Chronic Diseases: Overcoming Impediments to Prevention and Control. *JAMA*. 2004; 291:2616-2622.

11. Yasnoff, WA, et. al. A consensus action agenda for achieving the national health information infrastructure. *J. Am. Med. Inform. Assoc*. 2004; 11:332-338.

12. American Red Cross Museum. Available at: www.redcross.org/museum/history/brief_a.asp. Accessed April 23, 2007.

13. Edelman, R. NGOs approach parity in credibility with business and government in U.S. Available at: www.edelman.com/edelmannewsroom/releases/6477.html. Accessed April 2002.

CHAPTER 3

1. Carter J. *The Virtues of Aging*. New York, NY: Library of Contemporary Thought; 1998.

2. Brundtland GH. Speech on burden of disease concept at Hopitaux Universitaires de Geneve; December 15, 1998.

3. Alliance for Aging Research. Medical Never-Never Land Ten Reasons Why America is Not Ready for the Coming Age Boom. February 2002.

4. Manton KG, Corder LS, Stallard E. Monitoring changes in the health of the U.S. elderly populations: correlates with biomedical research and clinical innovations. *FASEB J*. 1997;11:923-930.

5. Havens B. *Improving the Health of Older People. A World View*. Oxford University Press; 1990.

6. Hobbs FB, Damon BL, eds. 65+ in the United States. Washington, DC: US Bureau of the Census; 1996.

7. Biomedical Innovations, Baby Boomers and Aging. *The Pfizer Journal*. 1999; 3:1, 5-6.

8. National Center for Health Statistics. 2000.

9. Valliant GE, Meyer SE, Mukamal K, Soldz S. Are social supports in late midlife a cause or result of successful physical aging? *Psychol Med*. 1998; 28:1159-1168.

10. Strawbridge WJ, Cohen RD, Shema SJ, Kaplan GA. Successful aging: predictors and associated activities. *Am J Epidemiol*.1996;144:135-141.

11. Vita AJ, Terry RB, Hubert HB, Fries JF. Aging, health risks, and cumulative disability. *NEJM*. 1998;339:481-482.

12. Pardes H, Manton KG, Lander ES, Tolley HD, Ullian AD, Palmer H. Effects of medical research on health care and the economy. *Science*. 1999;283:36-37.

13. Alzheimer's Association. 1998 National public policy program to conquer Alzheimer's disease. Washington, DC: Alzheimer's Association; 1998.

14. Koppel R. Alzheimer's cost to U.S. business. Washington, DC: Alzheimer's Association; September 1998.

15. Hodes RJ, Cahan V, Pruzan M. The National Institute on Aging at its twentieth anniversary: achievements and promise of research on aging. *J Am. Geriatr Soc*. 1996;44:204-206.

16. Penninx BW, Leveille S, Ferrucci L, et al. Exploring the effect of depression on physical disability: longitudinal evidence from the established populations for epidemiologic studies of the elderly. *Am J Public Health*. 1999; 89:1346-1352.

17. Kane RA, Kane RL, Ladd RC. *The Heart of Long-Term Care*. New York, NY: Oxford University Press;1998.

18. Meek PD. McKeithan K, Schumock GT. Economic considerations in Alzheimer's disease. *Pharmacotherapy*. 1998;18:68-73.

19. Freiman M, Brown E. *Special Care Units in Nursing Homes—Selected Characteristics, 1996*. Rockville, Md: Agency for Health Care Policy and Research; 1999. MEPS Research Findings #6. AHCPR Publication No. 99-0017; January 1999.

20. American Association of Retired Persons (AARP). Fitness: do you make physical activity an integral part of your daily routine? Available at: http://www.aarp.org/confacts/health/fitness.html. Accessed   September 13, 1999.

21. Fantl JA, Newman DK, Colling J, et al. Urinary incontinence in adults: acute and chronic management. Clinical Practice Guideline Number 2 (1996 Update). Rockville, MD: Agency for Health Care Policy and Research; 1996. AHCPR Publication No. 97-0682.

22. Perls TT. Centenarians prove the compression of morbidity hypothesis, but what about the rest of us who are genetically less fortunate? *Med Hypotheses*. 1997;49:405-407.

23. Shalala D. The United States Senate Special Committee on Aging. Long Term Care for the 21st Century: A Common Sense Proposal to Support Family Caregivers. Testimony before the United States Special Committee on Aging: March 23, 1999. Available at: http://www.senate.gov/~aging/hr29.htm. Accessed October 4, 1999.

24. Administration Association for Homes and Services for the Aging (AAHSA). Nursing homes [fact sheet]. Available at: http://www.aahsa.org/public/nursbkg.htm. Accessed June 16, 1999.

25. Day, JC. Population projections of the United States by Age, Sex, Race, and Hispanic Origin: 1995 to 2050. Current Population Reports. Washington DC: US Department of Commerce; Economics and Statistics Administration; US Bureau of the Census; February 1996. Publication No. P25-1130;12.

26. 1994 Green Book. Overview of Entitlement Programs. Committee on Ways

and Means, U.S. House of Representatives. Washington, DC; July 15, 1994. [Appendix B: Health Status, Insurance, Expenditures of the Elderly, and Background data on Long-Term Care]. Available at: http://bappend.txt at aspe.os.dhhs.gov. Accessed August 24, 1999.

27. Kemper P, Murtaugh CM. Lifetime use of nursing home care. *N Eng J Med*. 1991;324:595-600.

28. National Partnership for Women and Families. When you become a parent to your parents: finding the balance [press release]. August 10, 1999. Available at: http://www.nationalpartnership.org/news/pressreleases/1999/081099.htm. Accessed October 4, 1999.

29. Bishop CE. Where are the missing elders? The decline in nursing home use, 1985 and 1995. *Health Aff*. 1999;18:146-155.

30. Van Nostrand JF, Clark RF, Romoren TI. Nursing home care in five nations. *Aging Int*. 1993:1-5.

31. New environments for mature living. *The Pfizer Journal*. Volume 3. Number 3. 1999;3:3.

32. American Health Care Association (AHCA). Survey finds boomers headed for financial disaster in golden years [press release]..Available at: http://www.ahca.org/brief/nr990407.htm. Accessed September 27, 1999.

33. American Association of Homes and Services for the Aging (AAHSA). Long-Term Care Financing [Backgrounder]. Washington, DC: AAHSA; 1999. Available at: http://www.aahsa.org/public/ltfinbkg.htm. Accessed September 1, 1999.

34. Agency for Health Care Policy and Research. *ACHPR Research on Long-Term Care*. Available at: http://www.ahcpr.gov/research/longtrm1.htm. Accessed: August 30, 1999.

35. Reschovsky JD. The roles of Medicaid and economic factors in the demand for nursing home care. *Health Serv Res*. 1998;33:787-813.

CHAPTER 4

1. Dean, DJ. Every Women's Health in the New Millennium. *The Pfizer Journal*. 2001:5;1;100.

2. Seventeen Magazine. Web site questionnaire, October 2000. www.seventeen.com.

3. Cyranowski JM, Frank E, Young E, Shear MK. Adolescent onset of the gender difference in lifetime rates of major depression: a theoretical model. *Arch Gen Psychiatry*. 2000; 57:21-27.

4. In Harm's Way: Suicide in America. NIMH publication No. 01-4594. Available at: www.nimh.nih.gov/publicat/harmsway.cfm. Accessed April 4, 2001.

5. The Numbers Count. NIMH publication No. 01-4584. Available at: www.nimh.nih.gov. Accessed April 27, 2001.

6. Weisman CS. Women's health in perspective. In: *Women's Primary Care*. New York, NY: McGraw-Hill; 2000.

7. Hewitt S. *Creating a Life: Professional Women and the Quest for Children*. New York, NY: Miramax; 2002.

8. American Society for Reproductive Medicine. www.asrm.org. 2003.

9. Data Brief on Women and HIV/AIDS: The National Facts. Center for Women Policy Studies, Washington DC. Updated regularly.

10. Jacobs Institute of Women's Health. Guidelines for counseling women on the management of menopause. February 2000.

11. American Cancer Society. Breast cancer facts and figures 1996. Available at: www.cancer.org. Accessed: April 24, 2001.

12. The National Women's Health Information Center. Older Women's Health Priorities. Available at: www.4woman.gov. Accessed 24 April 2001.

13. Older Women's League (OWL). Osteoporosis: a challenge for midlife and older women. Available at: www.owl-national.org. Accessed 24 April 2001.

14. Arthritis Foundation. Women and arthritis. Available at: ww.intelihealth.com. Accessed: April 27 2001.

15. Older Women's League. Women and heart disease: a neglected epidemic. Available at: www.owl-national.org. Accessed 24 April, 2001.

16. Arno P, Levine C, Memmott M. The economic value of informal caregiving. Health Aff. 1999: 18;182-188.

17. The Commonwealth Fund 1998 Survey of Women's Health. Fact Sheet: Informal Caregiving. May 1999. Available at: www.cmwf.org.

18. Guralnik JM, Leveille SG, Hirsch R, et al. The impact of disability in older women. JAMWA. Summer 1997;52:113-120.

19. U.S. Census Bureau, population division. Available at: www.census.gov. Accessed 17 April 2001.

20. National Institutes of Health, Osteoporosis and Related Bone Diseases National Resource Center. Osteoporosis Overview. Available at: www.osteo.org/osteo.html. Accessed 10 June 2001.

21. NHLBI. Heart Disease & Women: Are You at Risk? NIH publication No. 98-3654. August 1998.

22. Surgeon General. Physical activity and health. Centers for Disease Control. Available at: http://www.cdc.gov. Accessed March 30, 2001.

23. Mosca L, Manson E, Sutherland SE, et al. Cardiovascular disease in women: a statement for healthcare professionals from the American Heart Association. Circulation. 1997; 96:2468-2482.

24. American Heart Association. Women, Heart Disease and Stroke Statistics. 2000. Available at: http://www.americanheart.org.

25. American Lung Association. Facts about lung cancer. Available at http://www.lungusa.org/diseases/lungcan.html. Accessed January 23, 2001.

26. American Cancer Society. Breast cancer: what is it? Available at http://www3.cancer.org. Accessed January 23, 2001.

27. Surgeon General. Women and Smoking: Centers for Disease Control. Available at: http://www.cdc.gov. Accessed March 29, 2001.

28. Women Hold Up Half the Sky. NIMH publication No. 99-4607. Available at: http://www.nimh.nih.gov. Accessed December 22, 2000.

29. Depression: What Every Woman Should Know. NIMH publication No 00-4779. August 2000. Available at: http://www.nimh.nih.gov. Accessed December 2, 2000.

30. Parry BL, Haynes P. Mood disorders and the reproductive cycle. *The Journal of Gender-Specific Medicine*. 2000;3:53-58.

31. Kilpatrick DG, Edmunds CN, Seymour A. Rape in America: A Report to the Nation. National Victim Center: 1992.

32. *Sexually Transmitted Diseases Fact Sheet*. National Institute of Allergy and Infectious Diseases. Available at: http://www.niaid.nih.gov. Accessed March 27, 2001.

33. Woman-Focused Response to HIV/AIDS. A Publication of the National AIDS Fund in collaboration with the Center for Women Policy Studies.

34. Woods N, Laffrey S, Duffy M, et al. Being healthy: women's images. *Advances in Nursing Science*. 1988;1:36-46.

35. Collins KS, Schoen C, Joseph S, et al. Health concerns across a woman's lifespan. The Commonwealth Fund 1998 Survey of Women's Health, May 1999.

36. A Profile of Caregiving in America. *The Pfizer Journal*. Fall 1997.

CHAPTER 5

1. Cohen JL. Human Population: The Next Half Century. *Science*. November 14, 2003:1172-1175.

2. Alliance for Aging Research. Medical Never-Never Land Ten Reasons Why America is Not Ready for the Coming Age Boom." February 2002.

3. Magee M. and D'Antonio M. *The Best Medicine*. New York: St. Martin's Press; 2001.

4. Nash D. Connecting with the New Health Care Consumer. New York:McGraw-Hill;2001.

5. Dishman E. Inventing Wellness Systems for Aging in Place. *Computer*. 2004;37:34-41.

6. Pew, RW and Van Hemel, SB eds. Technology for Adaptive Aging. Nat'l Research Council, 2003. Cited in Dishman E.

7. Massachusetts Institute of Technology Web site. Available at: http://architecture.mit.edu/house_n/. Accessed April 12, 2005.

8. University of Michigan Web site. Available at: http://www.eecs.umich.edu/~pollackm/. Accessed April 12, 2005.

9. University of Virginia Web site. Available at: http://marc.med.virginia.edu/projects_smarthomemonitor.html. Accessed April 15, 2005.

10. University of Rochester Web site. Available at: http://www.centerforfuturehealth.org/. Accessed April 12, 2005.

11. General Electric Web site. Available at: http://geglobalresearch.com/01_coretech/homeAssurance.shtml. Accessed April 12, 2005.

12. NASA Web site. Available at: http://science.nasa.gov/headlines/y2004/28oct_nanosensors.htm. Accessed April 12, 2005.

13. i.d.e.a.s., a spin-off of the Walt Disney Company, Web site. Available at: http://www.integrityarts.com/ideas.html. Accessed April 12, 2005.

14. Best Buy: Owner of eq-life. Available at: www.eq-life.com. Accessed April 12, 2005.

15. Philips Web site. Available at: http://www.medical.philips.com/main/products/telemonitoring/products/telemonitoring/. Accessed April 15, 2005.

16. Arno PS, Levine C, Memmott MM. The economic value of informal caregiving. *Health Aff.* 1999;18:182-188.

17. A Profile of Caregiving in America. *The Pfizer Journal.* Fall 1997.

18. Schultz R, O'Brien AT, Bookwala J, Fleissner K. Psychiatric and physical morbidity effects of dementia caregiving: prevalence, correlates, and causes. *Gerontologist.* 1995;35:771-91.

19. Grant I, Adler KA, Patterson TL, Dimsdale JE, Ziegler MG, Irwin MR. Health consequences of Alzheimer's caregiving transitions: effects of placement and bereavement. *Psychosom Med.* 2002;64:477-486.

20. First Annual Health Survey: Women Talk. National Women's Health Resource Center. May 2005.

21. Robinson JC. From managed care to consumer health insurance: the fall and rise of Aetna. *Health Aff* (Millwood). 2004;23:43-55.

22. Robinson JC. Reinvention of health insurance in the consumer era. *JAMA.* 2004;291:1880-1886.

CHAPTER 6

1. Magee M. Enduring Relationships in American Society. New York, NY: Yankelovich Partners, Omnibus Study. 1999.

2. Nash D. *Connecting with the New Health Care Consumer*: New York, NY: McGraw-Hill; 2001.

3. Magee M. Relationship Based Health Care in the United States, United Kingdom, Canada, Germany, South Africa and Japan. Annual Meeting, World Medical Association. Helsinki, Finland. September 11, 2003.

4. Magee, M and D'Antonion, M. *The Best Medicine*. 2003, New York :Spencer Books; 2003.

5. Magee, M. The Evolving Patient-Physician Relationship in America: From Paternalism to Partnership. New York, NY. Yankelovich Partners;1998.

6. Collins KS, Schoen C, Sondman DR. The Commonwealth Fund Survey of Physician Experience with Managed Care. Available at: www.omwf.org/health_care/physrvy.html. Accessed August 1998.

CHAPTER 7

1. Morrison RS, Meier DE. Palliative Care. *NEJM.* 2004;350:2582-2590.

2. Field MJ, Cassel CK, eds. Approaching death: improving care at the end of life. *National Academy Press.* Washington, DC. 1997. Cited in Morrison RS, Meier DE.

3. Quill TE. Perspectives on care at the close of life: initiating end-of-life

discussions with seriously ill patients: addressing the "elephant in the room." *JAMA*. 2000;284:2502-2507. Cited in Morrison RS, Meier DE.

4. Tulsky JA. Doctor-patient communication. In: Morrison RS, Meier DE, eds. *Geriatric palliative care*. New York: Oxford University Press; 2003:314-331. Cited in Morrison RS, Meier DE.

5. Steinhauser KE, Christakis NA, Clipp EC, McNeilly M, McIntyre L, Tulsky JA. Factors considered important at the end of life by patients, family, physicians, and other care providers. *JAMA*. 2000; 284:2476-2482. Cited in Morrison RS, Meier DE.

6. Fox E, et al. Evaluation of prognostic criteria for determining hospice eligibility in patients with advanced lung, heart, or liver disease. *JAMA*. 1999;282:1638-1648.

7. Prigerson, HG. Costs to Society of Family Caregiving for Patients With End Stage Alzheimer's Disease. *NEJM*. 349; 20; 1891-1892.

8. Schultz, R. et al. Psychiatric and physical morbidity effects of dementia caregiving: prevalence, correlates, and causes. Gerontologist 1995; 35: 771-91.

9. Schultz, R. et al. Caregiving as a risk factor for morbidity. The Caregiver Health Effects Study *JAMA*. 1999: 282; 2215-9.

10. Schultz, R. et al. End-of-Life Care and the Effects of Bereavement on Family Caregivers of Persons with Dementia. *NEJM*. 349; 20: 1936-42.

11. Grant I, et al. Health Consequences of Alzheimer's Caregiving Transitions: Effects of Placement and Bereavement. *Psychosom Med*. 2002; 64: 477-86.

12. Ory, MG., Et al. Prevalence and impact of caregiving: a detailed comparison between dementia and non-dementia caregivers. *Gerontologist*.1999; 39: 177-85.

CHAPTER 8

1. MetLife, National Alliance for Caregiving. Miles Away: The MetLife Study of Long-Distance Caregiving, July 2004.

2. National Alliance for Caregiving, AARP, MetLife. Caregiving in the U.S., April 2004. Cited in MetLife, National Alliance for Caregiving. Miles Away: The MetLife Study of Long-Distance Caregiving, July 2004.

3. Shellenbarger S. When Elderly Loved Ones Live Far Away: The Challenge of Long-Distance Care. *The Wall Street Journal*. July 29, 2004.

4. Lederman S. Private communication, 2005.

5. National Center on Elder Abuse. Reports of Domestic Elder Abuse. Available at: http://www.elderabusecenter.org/pdf/basics/fact1.pdf. Accessed February 28, 2005.

6. Lachs MS, Williams CS, O'Brien S, Pillemer KA, Charlson ME. The mortality of elder abuse. *JAMA*. 1998;280:428-443. National Academies of Sciences. Bonnie R, Wallace R, eds. Elder abuse: abuse, neglect, and exploitation in an aging America. Washington, D.C.: National Academy Press, 2002.

7. Lachs MS, Pillemer K. Abuse and neglect of elderly persons. *NEJM*. 1995;333:437.

8. Lachs MS, Pillemer K. Elder abuse. *The Lancet*. 2004;364:1263-1272.

CHAPTER 9

1. Getting Excited About the Technology Wave. Heath Politics Blog. January 4 2007. Available at: http://blog.healthpolitics.org/public/item/156722

2. Chen HY et al NEJM, "Five gene signature in non- small-cell lung cancer", 356:15, 1581-1583

3. CAST Web site. CAST sponsors. Available at: http://www.agingtech.org/sponsors.aspx.

4. CAST Web site. Imagine – the Future of Aging video. Available at: http://www.agingtech.org/imagine_video.aspx.

5. Dash E. Wall Street Senses Opportunities in Health Care Savings Accounts. *The New York Times*. January 20, 2006; A1.

6. UnitedHealth Group News Release. "Exante Financial Services Introduces Consumer Health Investment Options." November 7, 2005. Available at: http://www.unitedhealthgroup.com/news/rel2005/1107Exante.htm.

7. Blue Cross Blue Shield Health Issues News Release. "Blue Cross And Blue Shield Companies To Develop Bank." December 5, 2005. Available at: http://bcbshealthissues.com/proactive/newsroom/release.vtml?id=189255.

8. Yasnoff WA, Humphreys BL, Overhage JM, et al. A consensus action agenda for achieving the national health information infrastructure. *J Am Med Inform Assoc*. 2004;11:332-338.

9. National Committee on Vital and Health Statistics. Information for Health: A Strategy for Building the National Health Information Infrastructure. November 15, 2001. Available at: http://www.Ncvhs.hhs.gov/nhiilayo.pdf. Accessed January 19, 2004. Cited in Yasnoff WA, Humphreys BL, Overhage JM, et al.

10. Flynn LJ. Some Worries as San Francisco Goes Wireless. *The New York Times*. April 10, 2006. C5.

11. Gnatek T. Technology: Services. *The New York Times*. May 3, 2006.

12. Dash E, Belson K. Ring Up My Bill, Please; Mobile Payment Via Cellphone. *The New York Times*. March 21, 2006. C1.

CHAPTER 10

1. Detmer DE. "Getting to a 'Smarter' Health Information System: Legislative Proposals to Promote the Adoption of Electronic Health Records (EHRs)." Testimony Before the Committee on Energy and Commerce, Subcommittee on Health. March 16, 2006.

2. Expert Panel. "Personal Health Records and Electronic Health Records: Navigating the Intersection." Bethesda, MD. September 28-29, 2006.

3. Alliance for Aging Research. *Medical Never-Never Land Ten Reasons Why America is Not Ready for the Coming Age Boom*. February 2002.

4. Nash D, Manfredi MP, Bozarth B, Howell S. Connecting with the New Health Care Consumer. New York:McGraw-Hill Publishing Co; 2000.

5. Dishman E. Inventing Welless Systems for Aging in Place. *Computer*.

2004;37:31-34.

6. Hillestad R. Can Electronic Medical Record Systems Transform Health Care? *Health Affairs*. 2005;24:1103-1117.

7. Tang PC, Ash JS, Bates DW, Overage JM, Sands DZ. Personal Health Records: Definitions, Benefits, and Strategies for Overcoming Barriers to Adoption. *J Am Med Inform Assoc*. 2006;13:121-126.

8. Magee M. *Health Politics: Power, Populism and Health*. New York. Spencer Books. 2005.

9. Magee M. The Re-Emergence of Home Health Care: A Holistic Response to Aging and Consumer Empowerment in Medicine of the Person. Cox, J., Campbell AV and Fulford (eds). Jessica Kingsley Publishers, UK.

10. Magee M. "Turning Silos to Vapor: How the New Health Populism Will Transform Medicine As We Know It." Speech to the American Medical Association Presidents' Forum. Washington DC. March 12, 2006.

CHAPTER 11

1. Magee M, D'Antonio M. *The Best Medicine*. New York: Spencer Books; 2001.

2. Magee M. Relationship Based Health Care in the United States, United Kingdom, Canada, Germany, South Africa, and Japan. Presented at the World Medical Association Annual Meeting. Helsinki, Finland. September 11, 2003.

3. Haynes RB. *Determinants of compliance: the disease and the mechanics of treatment*. Baltimore: Johns Hopkins University Press; 1979.

4. World Health Organization. Adherence to Long-Term Therapies: Evidence for action. 2003. Available at: http://www.who.int/chronic_conditions/adherencereport/en/.

5. American Medical Association. The Patient's Role in Improving Adherence. Available at: http://www.ama-assn.org/ama/pub/article/12202-8427.html. Accessed October 21, 2004.

6. Magee M. Attacking Chronic Diseases in Developing Countries. Available at: http://www.healthpolitics.com/program_info.asp?p=prog_55. Accessed October 21, 2004.

7. Family Medicine NetGuide. Patient Adherence Explained. Available at: http://www.fmnetguide.com/vo2iss1/feature.html. Accessed October 21, 2004.

8. Pfizer Clear Health Communication Initiative 2003-2004.

CHAPTER 12

1. National Medical Association Convention. New York. July 25, 2005.

2. Magee M, D'Antonio M. *The Best Medicine*. New York: St. Martins Press/Spencer Books. New York. 2000.

3. Dishman E. Inventing Wellness Systems for Aging in Place. Computer. 2004;37:31-34.

4. Pew, RW and Van Hemel, SB, eds. Technology for Adaptive Aging. Nat'l Research Council, 2003. Cited in Dishman E.

5. Magee M. The Emergence of Home-Centered Health Care—Part II: Turning Visions into Reality. Available at: http://www.healthpolitics.com/archives.

asp?previous=home_health2&bhcp=1.

6. Lenfant, C. 2003. Clinical research to clinical practice—Lost in translation. *NEJM*. 2003;349:868-74.

7. Belden Russonello & Stewart, for Alliance for Aging Research. Great expectations: Americans' views on aging-Results of a national survey on aging research. Washington, DC: Alliance for Aging Research. 2001.

8. Adams K, Corrigan JM, eds. *Priority areas for national action: Transforming health care quality*. Washington, DC: National Academy Press;2003.

9. Schwartz K and Vilquin JT. Building the translational highway: Toward new partnerships between academia and the private sector. *Nature Medicine*. 2003; 9:493-5.

10. National Committee for Quality Assurance. The state of managed care quality. Washington, D.C.: National Committee for Quality Assurance. 1997.

11. National Committee for Quality Assurance. The state of managed care quality. Washington, D.C.: National Committee for Quality Assurance. 1999.

12. Awtry, E.H., Loscalzo, J. Aspirin. *Circulation*. 2000;101:1206-18.

13. National Registry of Myocardial Infarction. NMRI 4 quarterly data report 2002. San Francisco: Genentech;2002.

14. National Committee for Quality Assurance. The state of health care quality. Washington, D.C.: National Committee for Quality Assurance. 2002.

15. Magee M. Relationship Based Health Care in the United States, United Kingdom, Canada, Germany, South Africa and Japan. Annual Meeting, World Medical Association. Helsinki, Finland. September 11, 2003.

16. Montaner JSG, O'Shaughnessy MV, et al. Industry-sponsored clinical research: A double-edged sword. *Lancet*. 2001;358:1893-1895.

17. Giorganni, S., ed. Bench, bedside, and beyond: clinical research at the crossroads. *The Pfizer Journal*. 2002;6(3):29.

18. United States Senate Joint Economic Committee. The Benefits of Medical Research and the Role of the NIH. Washington, DC: United States Senate Joint Economic Committee. 2002.

19. MedBiquitous Web site. Mission and Scope. Available at: http://www.medbiq. org/about_us/mission/index.html. Accessed August 11, 2005.

20. Fischhoff B, Bostrom A, and Quadrel MJ. Risk perception and communication. *Annual Review of Public Health*. 1993;14:183-203.

21. Robinson JC. Reinvention of health insurance in the consumer era. *JAMA*. 2004; 291:1880-1886.

22. Magee M. Clinical Research at a Critical Juncture. Available at: http://www. healthpolitics.com/archives.asp?previous=prog_16. Accessed August 11, 2005.

23. Hibernia College Web site. Available at: http://www.hiberniacollege.net/ Default.aspx?tabid=1337. Accessed August 11, 2005.

CHAPTER 13

1. Lewin ME and Altman S. *America's Health Care Safety Net: Intact but*

Endangered. Washington DC. National Academy Press.

2. Hadley J and Holahan J. The Kaiser commission on Medicaid and the Uninsured. Who pays and how much? The cost of caring for the uninsured. The Urban Institute. February 2003.

3. World Health Organization Assesses the World's Health Systems [news release on World Health Organization Web site]. Available at: http://www.who.int/whr/2000/media_centre/press_release/en/print.html/html. Accessed November 30, 2004.

4. Committee on Assuring the Health of the Public in the 21st Century, Institute of Medicine. The Future of the Public's Health in the 21st Century. 2002. Available at: http://www.iom.edu/report.asp?id=4304. Accessed November 30, 2004.

5. Isaacs SL, Schroeder SA. Class—the ignored determinant of the nation's health. *NEJM*. 2004;351;1137-42.

6. Williams DR. Race and health: trends and policy implications. In: Auerbach JA, Krimgold BD, eds. Income, socioeconomic status, and health: exploring the relationships. Washington, D.C.: National Policy Association, 2001:70. Cited in Isaacs SL, Schroeder SA.

7. U.S. Census Bureau. Poverty in the United States, 1997. Available at: http://www.census.gov/prod/3/98pubs/p60-201.pdf. Accessed November 30, 2004. Cited in Isaacs SL, Schroeder SA.

8. McDonough P, Duncan GJ, Williams DR, House J. Income dynamics and adult mortality in the United States, 1972 through 1989. *Am J Public Health*. 1997;87:1476-83. Cited in Isaacs SL, Schroeder SA.

9. Health, United States. Hyattsville, Md.: National Center for Health Statistics, 2002:198. (DHHS publication no. (PHS) 2002-1232.) Cited in Isaacs SL, Schroeder SA.

10. Pratt M, Macera CA, Blanton C. Levels of physical activity and inactivity in children and adults in the United States: current evidence and research issues. *Med Sci Sports Exerc*. 1999;31:Suppl:S527-S533. Cited in Isaacs SL, Schroeder SA.

11. Davey Smith G, Blane D, Bartley M. Explanations for socio-economic differentials in mortality: evidence from Britain and elsewhere. *Eur J Public Health*. 1994;4:131-44. Cited in Isaacs SL, Schroeder SA.

12. McGinnis JM, Williams-Russo P, Knickman JR. The case for more active policy attention to health promotion. *Health Aff* (Millwood) 2002;21(2):78-93. Cited in Isaacs SL, Schroeder SA.

13. Fronstin P. Sources of health insurance and characteristics of the uninsured: analysis of the March 2005 current population survey. Issue brief. No. 287. Washington, D.C.: Employee Benefits Research Institute, 2005. Available at http://www.ebri.org/pdf/briefspdf/EBRI_IB_11-20051.pdf.

14. Blumenthal, D. Employer-Sponsored Health Insurance in the United States—Origins and Implications. *New England Journal of Medicine*, 355:1. July 6, 2006.

15. Gladwell, M. The Risk Pool. *The New Yorker*. August 28, 2006.

16. Thomasson M. From sickness to health: the twentieth century development of U.S. health insurance. *Explorations in Economic History,* 2002:32;233-53.

17. Appleby J, Silke Carty S. Ailing GM looks to scale back generous health benefits. *USA Today.* June 23, 2005:B1.

18. Chirba-Martin MA, Brennan TA. The critical role of ERISA in state health reform. *Health Aff* (Millwood)1994;13(2):142-56.

19. The impact of the erosion of retiree health benefits on workers and retirees. Issue brief. No. 279. Washington, D.C.: Employee Benefits Research Institute;2005. Available at http://www.ebri.org/publications/ib/index. cfm?fa=ibDisp&content_id=3497.

20. Harris RO. A sacred trust. New York: New American Library, 1966.

21. Freudenheim M. A new worry for investors: retirees' medical benefits. *The New York Times.* July 25, 2005: C3.

CHAPTER 14

1. AllBusiness.com. Health Care Reform: Déjà Vu All Over Again. September 2002. Available at: http://www.allbusiness.com/periodicals/article/274229-1. html.

2. Callaway D. GM Fears Cast Long Shadow. Marketwatch.com. November 17, 2005.

3. O'Dell J. Ford Unveils Wide Job Cuts. Los Angeles Times. January 24, 2006:A1.

4. Webster P. US big businesses struggle to cope with health-care costs. *The Lancet.* 2006;367:101-102.

5. Freudenheim M, Williams Walsh M. The Next Retirement Time Bomb. *The New York Times.* December 11, 2005:B1.

6. GASB-OPEB Web page. Frequently Asked Questions. Available at: http:// gasb-opeb.com/faq.htm.

7. Standard & Poor's Web site. Available atL http://www2.standardandpoors. com/servlet/Satellite?pagename=sp/Page/HomePg&r=1&l=EN.

8. Mercer Human Resource Consulting. Addressing the Challenges and Opportunities. Available at: http://www.mercerhr.com/summary.jhtml?idCo ntent=1143390&originUrl=/knowledgecenter/home.jhtml%3Frl%3D.

9. White House News Release. Fact Sheet: America's Ownership Society: Expanding Opportunities. Available at: http://www.whitehouse.gov/news/ releases/2004/08/20040809-9.html.

10. Himmelstein DU, Warren E, Thorne D, Woolhandler S. Illness and injury as contributors to bankruptcy. *Health Affairs Web Exclusive.* February 2, 2005.

11. Kennedy EM. *In Critical Condition: The Crisis in America's Health Care.* New York: Simon and Schuster;1972.

12. Merlis M. "Family Out-of-Pocket Spending for Health Services." New York: Commonwealth Fund;June 2002.

13. NPR/Kaiser Family Foundation/Kennedy School of Government. "National Survey on Health Care (chartpack)." June 2002.

CHAPTER 15

1. Weissman DE. Decision making at a time of crisis near the end of life. *JAMA*. 2004;292:1738-1743.

2. Lamont EB, Christakis NA. Prognostic disclosure to patients with cancer near the end of life. *Ann Intern Med*. 2001;134:1096-1105. Cited in Weissman DE.

3. Ahronheim JC, Morrison RS, Baskin SA, et al. Treatment of the dying in the acute care hospital. *Arch Intern Med*. 1996;156:2094-2100. Cited in Weissman DE.

4. McCahill LE, Krouse RS, Chu DZJ, et al. Decision making in palliative surgery. *J Am Coll Surg*. 2002;195:411-423. Cited in Weissman DE.

5. Fallowfield LJ, Jenkins VA, Beveridge HA. Truth may hurt but deceit hurts more: communication in palliative care. *Palliat Med*. 2002;16:297-303. Cited in Weissman DE.

6. Elisabeth Kubler-Ross Web site. Available at: www.elisabethkublerross.com. Accessed May 19, 2005.

7. Cancer Survivors Web site. Available at: http://www.cancersurvivors.org/Coping/end%20term/stages.htm. Accessed May 19, 2005.

8. Prigerson HG, Jacobs SC. Caring for bereaved patients: "all the doctors just suddenly go." *JAMA*. 2001;286:1369-1376.

CHAPTER 16

1. Donelan K, et al. Challenged to care: Informal caregivers in a changing health system. *Health Affairs*. 2002;21:222-231.

2. Magee M, D'Antonio M. *The Best Medicine*. New York, NY; Saint Martin's Press; 1993.

3. Emanuel EJ, Emanuel LL. The promise of a good death. *The Lancet*. 1998;351(suppl2):S1121-A1129. Quoted in Teno JM et al.

4. Teno JM, et al. Family perspectives on end-of-life care at the last place of care. *JAMA*. 2004;291:88-93.

5. Saunders C. Care of patients suffering from terminal disease at St. Joseph's Hospice, Hackney, London. *Nursing Mirror*. 1964;vii-x.

Fox E, et al. Evaluation of prognostic criteria for determining hospice eligibility in patients with advanced lung, heart, or liver disease. *JAMA*.